Old and Poor

Old and Poor

A Critical Assessment of the
Low-Income Elderly

William F. Clark
Anabel O. Pelham
Marleen L. Clark

Lexington Books
D.C. Heath and Company/Lexington, Massachusetts/Toronto

The statements contained in this book are solely those of the authors and do not necessarily reflect the views or policies of the Health Care Financing Administration or of the State of California. Research for this volume was partially supported by HCFA Grant No. 11–P–97553/9–04–MSSP.

Portions of Chapter 7 are adapted from Anabel O. Pelham and William F. Clark, "Widowhood Among Low-Income Racial and Ethnic Groups in California," *Widows, Volume II, North America,* Helena Z. Lopata (ed.), Durham, N.C.: Duke University Press, © 1987.

For Marisol and Giselle, for all the CSS participants
who so willingly answered questions,
for Celia and Diane, who work for productive and positive aging.

Library of Congress Cataloging-in-Publication Data

Clark, William F.
   Old and poor: a critical assessment of the low-income elderly/
by William F. Clark, Anabel O. Pelham, Marleen L. Clark.
      p.   cm.
Bibliography: p.
Includes index.
ISBN 0–669–11078–7 (alk. paper)
   1. Aged—United States—Economic conditions—Case studies.   2. Old
age assistance—United States—Case studies.   3. Aged—Care—United
States—Case studies.   4. Cost and standard of living—United
States—Case studies.   I. Pelham, Anabel O.   II. Clark, Marleen L.
III. Title.
HV1461.C53   1988
362.6′ 0973—dc19   88–858
                                                                                          CIP

Published simultaneously in Canada
Printed in the United States of America
International Standard Book Number: 0–669–11078–7
Library of Congress Catalog Card Number 85–40456

The paper used in this publication meets the minimum requirements of American National Standard for Information Sciences—Permanence of Paper for Printed Library Materials, ANSI Z39.48–1984. ∞™

89 90 91 92 8 7 6 5 4 3 2

Contents

Illustrations

Tables

1
Introduction

Old and Poor

Nearly 3.5 million people in the United States are poor and old (U.S. Census 1987b). Each day, about sixteen hundred people sixty-five years old enter this group. While they are the major focus of public programs that annually cost billions of dollars, we know very little about their circumstances. The purpose of this book is to describe those circumstances so that public policies may better meet their needs.

Our primary information source is the California Senior Survey (CSS). The CSS was a longitudinal study of two thousand Medicaid elders carried out from 1980 to 1983. Research assistants collected detailed information through face-to-face interviews, to which were added data from Medicaid and Medicare records. Interview data covered demographic information, physical and mental functional status, family situation, services use, and health-related questions. From this rich data base, combined with the Medicare and Medicaid information, a fairly complete image emerges of the old and poor and their circumstances. To this quantitative depiction we add vignettes based on open-ended interviews with selected CSS respondents. These stories provide the human details missing from the numerical data and complete our picture of the old and poor. Our intention throughout this volume is to portray as accurately as possible the situation of the poor elderly without glorifying or "gore-ifying" their circumstances.

We also look at what happens to them as they go through the "continuum of care." This notion of a "continuum of care" stems from social planners and program advocates who see social and health services arrayed in a configuration to meet the least severe needs (e.g., socialization) to the most severe needs (e.g., institutionalization). This planning concept envisions all the "right" services in place and the aged person's ability to move from one point on the continuum to another. If the aged person cannot negotiate this movement by himself or herself, then enabling mechanisms, such as case management programs, should be in place to see that it does happen. This concept implies a unidirectional movement—that the elder goes from least to most severe. As we shall see in detail, actual movement patterns are quite different.

Understanding the actual movement patterns is crucial for planning and budgeting purposes. As resources become more scarce and intergenerational competition for them becomes more intense, problem areas should be well-defined and ameliorating policies specified as completely as possible. Chapter 6 discusses the concept of a continuum of care and services use in full detail.

To provide a context for our findings we first examine the concept of "poverty" and how it is now measured by the U.S. government.

The Concept of Poverty Revisited

Over the last one hundred years in the United States, the concept of poverty has been discovered and rediscovered several times, most notably twenty years ago with the War on Poverty. President Lyndon Johnson, based on ideas developed by President Kennedy, announced a "war on poverty" in 1964. The armamentarium for this war consisted of a set of new federally funded programs housed in the specially created Office of Economic Opportunity. Such activities as the Jobs Corps, Head Start, and community action programs—guided by the maxim of "maximum feasible participation"—began in the mid-sixties.

After a decade of struggle and intense activity, Congress cut off funding for OEO and the war was officially over in 1974. Congress eliminated funding for OEO because of competing fiscal demands for another war—Vietnam—and because of the gradual political disillusionment generated by OEO's grassroots political efforts.

Each time poverty became a public debate focus, a conceptual problem accompanied the discussions. The conceptual problem is the cause of poverty—is it cultural or is it the structure of the economy? The culture of poverty argument, based on the work of Oscar Lewis, held that poverty affected the very personality of the poor and that the culture of poverty was familial and intergenerational (Lewis 1961).

The structuralist point of view saw poverty as an economic situation caused by lack of opportunities. At the end of the sixties, a consensus emerged that poverty was less a cultural trait than an economic condition (Aaron 1978). However, as James Paterson (1981) points out, one of the most useful analytic contributions stemming from these debates between the structuralist and cultural points of view was Michael Harrington's (1962) point: " . . . that an obdurate new poverty devasted certain deprived groups in American life. They were the aged, migrant workers, small farmers, non-whites, people with little education, and children in female-headed families."

As Paterson states in his carefully researched history of twentieth century American attitudes toward the poor, these groups have always been there and have always been poor but, because of Harrington, they became the center of much public interest.

To be in poverty means that a person does not have a cash income equivalent of three times the cost of an "Economy Food Plan." The Department of Agriculture first established this plan from its 1955 Survey of Food Consumption. It was later adopted by the Social Security Administration (SSA) in 1964 as the official poverty index for United States government programs and policies (Schulz 1985). It has been revised by Federal Interagency Committees in 1969 and 1980. The poverty thresholds are updated every year to reflect changes in the Consumer Price Index (CPI).

The initial Department of Agriculture food plan, the Low Cost Food Plan, was used until 1964 when it was replaced by the more restrictive Economy Food Plan, which in turn was revised in 1975 into the present Economy Food Plan (Applebaum 1977). The food budget from the food plan was multiplied by three since the Department of Agriculture estimated that food expenditures make up about one-third of money income after taxes. Even before its adoption by SSA, the index was the subject of much debate within academia and within Congressional hearing rooms. Depending on how an index was constructed, poverty as a national problem could take on either minimal or maximal proportions. Where to draw the poverty line ranged from "minimum subsistence" to "minimum comfort" (Applebaum 1977) and produced ranges of the number of U.S. households in poverty from 11 percent to 40 percent.

In reality, there exist two official poverty levels: one for the group aged fifteen years old to sixty-four years old and another for those sixty-five years old and over. In 1984, the threshold for a single person in the younger group was $5,400 and for a person in the older group it was $4,979, or 8 percent less. For a two-person household, the younger threshold was $6,973; for the older two-person household it was $6,282, and 11 percent difference.

The reason two poverty lines exist stems from the original concept of the Economy Food Plan. USDA analysts assumed that older healthy people have lower nutritional requirements than younger people. This means the elderly's poverty line is less because it reflects lower food costs. The Villers Foundation (1987) estimates that:

If the same poverty standard were applied to the elderly as is now used to measure poverty among other age groups, the number of elderly poor would increase by 450,000 to 700,000 jumping from 3.5 million under the current count to as high as 4.2 million. By the same token, the poverty rate for the elderly would increase from 12.6 percent (under the current discriminatory standard) to as high as 15.2 percent.

An important characteristic of the SSA poverty index is that it is an *absolute* measure that considers only what it takes to maintain a minimal diet. Once nutritional elements are defined, consumption preferences established, and prices set, the resultant costs are multiplied by three. The relative position of the poor is not accounted for. Through mass media, the poor are acutely aware of their status and their relative deprivation when compared to the lower and middle classes, let alone the upper classes. Attempts to set the poverty line in relation to median income levels, and thereby making the index a relative measure, have always failed.

Public Policies and Poverty in the Seventies

Public concerns of the seventies—Vietnam, inflation, and Watergate—did not leave much "policy space" for poverty issues. However, two significant events related to poverty did occur in the U.S. Congress in 1972: the defeat of the Family Assistance Plan (FAP) and the passage of the Supplemental Security Income (SSI) plan. The proliferation of anti-poverty programs in the sixties created the impression of a "welfare mess." Also, a real increase in the number of people on the major welfare program, Aid to Families with Dependent Children (AFDC), created a "welfare crisis." Given the ascendancy of the structuralist point of view, the consensus among the experts at the time, both conservative and liberal, favored some type of income maintenance policy. Specifically, most authorities favored a form of guaranteed cash income for all the poor. The debates about how exactly this would be carried out culminated in 1969 with Nixon's Family Assistance Plan which would have guaranteed all families with children a minimum of five hundred dollars per adult and three hundred dollars per child per year, or sixteen hundred dollars for a two-parent family of four (Paterson 1981). The Nixon proposal also contained a "workfare" section that required adult recipients to accept training or work or forego payments. After three years of particularly bitter Congressional debate among elected officials, welfare rights advocates, academics, welfare recipients, and program administrators, the FAP proposal was shelved. A combination of critics from the right, who did not believe in handing out cash to the "undeserving poor," and from the left, who thought the minimum was too little and who did not like the workfare aspects of FAP, created an unlikely coalition that ultimately killed FAP. The multitude of in-kind programs (eg., training, child care, food stamps, and Medicaid) remained as the principal public instruments against poverty.

The major exception to this in-kind approach was the Supplemental Security Income program, passed in 1972. SSI replaced Old Age Assistance, a grant-in-aid program established by the Social Security Act in 1935 to assist the aged, blind, and disabled through three separate programs. These three programs had been administered by the states for almost forty years. SSI, financed totally from federal general tax revenues and operated by the Social Security Administration, provided a national minimum income to eligible aged, blind, and disabled persons. Eligibility was based on need as determined by level of income, both earned and unearned, and resources. The national minimum amount and uniform federal eligibility regulations and guidelines eliminated many interstate inequities that had developed during the operation of the Old Age Assistance program. In addition to the SSI amount, a state could choose to supplement the federal payment. As of 1987, twenty-six states and the District of Columbia have such a plan (Villers Foundation 1987). In California this is known as the State Supplemental Payment (SSP). States may choose to administer their own supplemental payment program or elect for federal administration.

Initially, in 1972, the maximum federal payment was $130 per month. When the program actually began in 1974 the maximum was $140 for aged individuals and $210 for aged couples. In 1975, automatic cost-of-living increases were incorporated into the payment system (Rich and Baum 1984). During fiscal year 1982–1983, the maximum was $285.50 for an individual and $426.40 for a couple. As of 1 January 1987, the aged individual maximum was $340; for the aged couple, $510.

Structural reformists were able to secure passage of SSI but not FAP for a variety of reasons. First, SSI was a change—albeit a significant change—to an existing known program, Old Age Assistance, and not a brand-new concept such as a guaranteed cash income. Congress is, as are most of us, more comfortable with incremental changes than with making radical departures from the past. Secondly, with complete federal funding, it provided states with fiscal relief, because the Old Age Assistance program required some state financial participation through a matching formula. Congressional leaders from all political persuasions favored this. Thirdly, the federal administration of the program would allow either a reduction in the state and county welfare apparatus or a redirection of efforts into new areas. The opportunities this administrative shift created had broad political appeal. Fourth, the categories of people who would benefit from SSI were the "deserving poor"—the aged, blind, and disabled—and therefore did not offend anyone's sense of equity. Fifth and finally, the FAP debates were particularly intense and a tremendous amount of energy was expended by all parties between 1969 and 1972. To go away at the end without "doing something" about the welfare "mess" was difficult for all participants. The SSI program at least combined three separate programs, provided fiscal relief to the states, created a uniformly administered national program with national minimum payment levels, increased the amount of cash in the hands of some of the poor, and, philosophically, created a "revolutionary right to cash income" (Burke and Burke 1974). As a "second-best solution," SSI, in 1974, provided substantive assistance to 3.2 million individuals who received payments that totaled $365.1 million (U.S. Department of Health and Human Services 1984).

As of December 1985, the SSI program served 4.1 million people. Some 1.5 million were in the "aged" category and the remainder were made up of blind and disabled individuals. Of the blind and disabled, an additional 586,783 were over age sixty-four (25,489 blind and 561,294 disabled) (Kahn 1987).

In-Kind Transfers and Poverty

As the public programs for the poor grew during the seventies, some analysts began to place a value on the goods and services involved—the in-kind transfers—to determine what impact a valuation of them would have on poverty levels. For example, if the Medicare benefits an aged poor person received because of a hospital stay were treated as "income," how would that amount of money affect his or her poverty status? Thomas Smeeding (1982) undertook for the U.S. Census Bureau the most comprehensive estimations of the effects of these in-kind programs, the largest being Medicaid and Medicare. He found that, depending on how one values the goods and services, the poverty rate could fall from 14.7 percent (the 1979 rate that he used as a base) to 4.5 percent, a drop from 4 million elderly to a little more than 1 million. This is a classic example of "defining away the problem."

Although an interesting analytical approach to poverty, the logical conclusion to it would be that a poor person who is the sickest and most needy of services turns out to be the "richest." Ridiculous logic. Nonetheless, this argument about the value of in-kind transfers is still discussed, particularly in the context of intergenerational competition of resources (e.g., should more tax dollars go to children's programs or to programs for the elderly?). The U.S. Census Bureau continues to carry out technical analyses on the topic.

The Eighties and the "New Poverty"

The recession of 1982–1983, with its unemployment rates reaching over 20 percent, focused attention on a group of people who found themselves in poverty for the first time because of structural unemployment or demographics and social conditions. The structural unemployment came about because of the aging industrial infrastructure of some of the country's "smokestack" industries, such as steel manufacturing. Harrington (1984) tells of this situation with graphic details from the Monongahela Valley region of Pennsylvania and brings home the fact that, for many of us, poverty is just a paycheck away. With intense competition from abroad, unemployment is becoming a fact of life in many industries.

A concomitant social problem with unemployment is the lack of health insurance. The newly unemployed who lose their medical coverage may be ineligible for Medicaid because it is a means-tested program. In some states they may not qualify because they own their own homes. Only when the home is lost will the pauperization process be complete enough for a person to qualify for Medicaid in some states.

The other major group to make up the "new Poverty" are women. Diana Pearce (1978) first brought attention to this growing social and demographic trend in her study, "The Feminization of Poverty: Women, Work, and Welfare," in which she reported that poverty is rapidly becoming a female problem. She and a colleague, Harriette McAdoo, continued to report on this problem and in another study (1981) concluded that the poverty rate for female-headed households is six times that of male-headed households. A report by the California Commission on the Status of Women (1983) reviewed several studies and reiterated Pearce's point that two out of three adults in poverty are women. Another California report, carried out by Lieutenant Governor Leo McCarthy's Task Force on the Feminization of Poverty (1985), cited a study that said:

> Simply put, social and economic processes are taking place in which women are increasingly bearing the brunt of being poor in America. As one statistic revealed, 'All other things being equal, if the proportion of the poor who are in female-headed families were to increase at the same rate as it did from 1967 to 1977, they would comprise 100% of the poverty population by about the year 2000. [President's National Advisory Council on Economic Opportunity 1981]'

The social process that leads to this feminization of poverty is marital dissolution and minimal or no child-support payments. In 1981, 41 percent of the 8.4 million women supporting their children in households with absent fathers *did not have* a court-ordered child support award or a private agreement with absent fathers. For those mothers below the poverty level, 60 percent did not have a child support award (U.S. Census 1983a).

The economic trends that contribute to the feminization of poverty are the occupational segregation patterns that separate women from the better-paying jobs that men hold and wage differentials that show women earn 59 percent of the median male wage (U.S. Department of Labor 1982a). Because of past and present occupational trends, half of all women work in just twenty of the 440 recognized occupational categories, occupations where wages are significantly lower than in the male-dominated categories (Rubin 1981).

The significance of this phenomenon for our present purposes is that, although the recession of 1982–1983 precipitated large-scale unemployment, the economic recovery that followed provided the traditional cure for white male poverty—a job—but did nothing for female poverty. For males, poverty may be just a paycheck away, but for women, poverty is often just a man away because of divorce and/or no child support and a job market that shunts women into lower-paying jobs. As we shall see, the story of the OLD AND POOR is mainly about women and, given the demographic, social, and economic trends sketched above, future reports on this subject will continue to be mostly about women. If occupational segregation patterns persist, and if no corrective action is taken toward insuring payment of child support, an underclass of poor aged women will become a permanent feature of American society—an aged female lumpen. Although in chapter 12 we make policy recommendations affecting the aged poor, serious attention should be paid to the economic plight of younger women. Without treating the root causes of the problems, the effects will always be with us.

Although the aged per se are not part of the "new poverty" of the eighties, Harrington (1984) makes a useful distinction when he discusses the "poverties" that still exist in American society. There are the new poverties stemming from structural unemployment, related to international economic trends, and from marital dissolutions that coexist with the traditional obdurate poverties of, for example, Native Americans and the aged. What is significant about the aged's poverty in the eighties is not its type but its size—3.5 million—although, over the last three decades, the proportion of elderly who are impoverished has dropped dramatically. For example, in 1959, 35.2 percent of the elderly were poor; in 1970, it was 24.5 percent; and, in 1980, it was 15.7 percent (U.S. Congress 1982). In 1986, it was 12.4 percent (U.S. Census, 1987b). As the relative number of elderly below poverty has become smaller, the amount of public transfers to the elderly in general has grown to such a point as to cause serious debate over the intergenerational equity of such policies (Preston 1984). We certainly agree that poverty rates among groups of the nonaged are shockingly high (e.g., black children and married, middle-aged females of all races with absent spouses) and that these groups merit more financial assistance. We also believe our national priorities should be such as to allow for this additional assistance without taking away from gains already made by other groups. We discuss this question of national priorities more fully in chapter 12.

Although the relative proportion of elderly who live below the poverty line has been decreasing, the absolute number has remained over 3 million since 1972. The actual numbers have ranged from 3.1 million (1974) to 3.9 million (1980) to the present 3.5 million (1986), and it appears the United States will continue to have a sizeable group of long-term aged poor as long as it maintains current social and economic policies. As the pauperization process known as the "feminization of poverty" continues, more and more younger recruits will join the ranks of the "old and poor," so that we will see in the 1990s a group numbering well over 5 million.

Poverty and the Elderly in the Eighties

Some aspects of poverty, as it affects the aged, are worthy to note so that our general understanding is more complete.

About 90 Percent of the Aged Poor Are Totally
Dependent on Transfer Payments as Source of Income.

U.S. Census data show that only about 10 percent of the aged poor have any source of income from earnings, meager as they may be. Also, about 82 percent of the aged poor receive some level of payment from Social Security but, for 1984, only about 23 percent receive any payment from the Supplemental Security Income program (including those who also receive Social Security payments) (U.S. Census, table 11, 1985a). What this means is that the overwhelming majority of the aged poor have participated in the labor force during their lives or, in the case of widows and widowers, their spouses have participated. The aged poor, as our vignettes illustrate, are those individuals who have been the delivery truck drivers, the taxi cab drivers, the sales clerks, the seamstresses—all the low-end service occupations. After living at near-poverty their entire lives, they find themselves "retired into poverty." At the end of their working lives, or at the death of a spouse, they spend the next fifteen or twenty years of their lives—about 20 to 25 percent of their entire lives and about 25 to 30 percent of their adult lives—in "official" poverty. The traditional means of escaping poverty—marriage or a job—are not readily available to the aged poor, so their poverty status, with few exceptions, is permanent.

The overall picture of the aged poor then is not typically one of a sudden displacement from a middle-class economic situation to a lower class, but rather from a life-long low economic class to the lowest—totally dependent on governmental transfers without any other source of income.

Not One Means-Tested Program Reaches the Majority
of the Poor Elderly

The major means-tested programs (programs for which you have to prove your lack of means—cash or countable assets—to participate in their benefits) that affect the elderly are: SSI, food stamps, subsidized housing, and Medicaid (the governmental health insurance program for the poor of all ages). We have already pointed out the relatively low program participation in SSI, and additional U.S. Census data reveal that only about 28 percent of elderly householders below the poverty level participate in the food stamps program and 31 percent live in subsidized housing (U.S. Census 1983c).

Program statistics for Medicaid, as they relate to elderly households living below the poverty level, are more difficult to obtain. In 1982, Medicaid recipients sixty-five years old and older totaled 3,368,000 (Rich and Baum 1984), but not all were below the poverty level and about 623,300 were nursing home residents and not part of the noninstitutionalized population (Lloyd and Greenspan 1985).

The Villers Foundation report (1987), cited earlier, states that "only 36 percent of the noninstitutionalized elderly poor—only about one in three—have Medicaid protection." This comes about because of the situation in which eligibility, as a general rule, is tied to participation in the SSI program. As we already saw, the SSI program participation among the aged poor is low, which, by extension, affects the Medicaid program participation rate. In addition, because Medicaid is a state-administered program, some states stipulate restrictive eligibility criteria and have created a confusing array of categorical groups and income levels, which excludes many poor people of all ages (Brown 1984).

The exact level of SSI program participation is not certain. For example, when we examine U.S. Census tables, we estimate the participation rate to be 23 percent among the aged poor. Louis Harris and Associates (1986) estimates that 17 percent of the elderly below the poverty line report receiving SSI. The Villers Foundation (1987), citing U.S. Census Data, states that among elderly *households*—not individuals—only 32 percent participate in the SSI program. The Commonwealth Fund Commission's (1987) estimate of program participation is 34 percent. Whatever the "true" rate of participation, it is certainly low and we can safely say that less than half the poor elderly receive SSI payments.

For those who do receive SSI, its maximum benefit levels are below the poverty level (U.S. Department of Health and Human Services 1984; U.S. Census 1983b). For example, for 1987, the maximum Federal SSI benefit for an individual was 76 percent of the poverty threshold; for a couple, the benefit represented 90 percent of the threshold (Commonwealth Fund Commission 1987). As of 1 January 1985, only 20 percent of aged individuals and 23 percent of couples received the maximum monthly SSI payment, reflecting that a significant proportion of them also received social security benefits or other countable income (Kahn 1987).

Possible explanations for the low participation rate in SSI have to do with eligibility rules. One rule states that an individual can only have countable assets of eighteen hundred dollars and, for a couple, twenty-seven hundred dollars (as of 1987). The original ceilings, fixed in 1972, were fifteen hundred dollars and two thousand dollars for an individual and a couple.

Obviously, these ceilings have not kept up with inflation and potential program participants are excluded because of this lack of a correction for inflation.

Another rule deals with the reduction by one-third of benefits if the SSI recipient lives in the household of another for a full month and receives maintenance and support. The net effect of the reduction may mean to the recipient that it is not worth the administrative hassle—the transaction costs—to continue with the program or to make the initial contact with an intrusive welfare bureaucracy.

Most Aged Poor Are White Widows Living Alone
in a Metropolitan Area, Outside of a Poverty Area,
in Their Own Homes.

The story of poverty among the elderly is a woman's story—70 percent of the aged poor are female. This woman is also white by the sheer numbers involved (2 million) but the poverty rate among black females is almost three times as much as it is for the white female: 42.4 percent versus 15.1 percent (U.S. Census 1984a). Perhaps contrary to popular mythology, our "typical" poor old woman does not live in an inner-city hotel room but rather owns her own home in a metropolitan area outside of those census tracts which have more than 20 percent of the population below the poverty level.

Family Life, Family Interactions, and Family Helping
Patterns Among the Aged Poor Are Similar to Those
Found Among the General Elderly Population.

The family life we examine in some detail reveals a strong and helpful family structure, which mirrors those patterns found among the more affluent elderly. Whatever problems a lack of cash has created, poverty does not seem to affect family life among the aged poor. The amount of help provided by family members—mainly the spouse or daughter—to those who need it is impressive. On the whole, frequent contact and reciprocal behavior are very much alive and well among the aged poor and their families. As we see in chapter 9, this help and caring extends to when the elderly person is placed in a nursing home. This family life is in contrast to the social problems and ills that Moynihan (1965) found among the young poor and termed a "tangle of pathology."

We turn our attention now to the California Senior Survey and certain methodological considerations.

2
Methodological Considerations

California Senior Survey Sampling Strategy

The original purpose of the California Senior Survey was to act as a comparison group for a large research and demonstration project, the California Multipurpose Senior Services Project (MSSP). MSSP was a four-year, community-based, long-term care demonstration whose purpose was to generate information about effective ways to maintain the elderly at home and to avoid nursing home placements. The MSSP clients—the experimental group—were low-income elders, sixty-five and over, Medicaid (Medi-Cal in California) recipients and received the MSSP intervention of case management and additional services. We have reported the results of the MSSP demonstration elsewhere (Miller, Clark, and Clark 1985).

To determine the effects of the experimental intervention, a comparison group of similar individuals was formed, interviewed, and re-interviewed during the same period. This comparison group, known as the California Senior Survey, did not receive any services from MSSP but used, when needed, the existing set of services available to all low-income elderly in California.

The entire CSS consisted of three subsamples, which mirrored the MSSP's own subsamples and which are defined by the residential status of the participant at point of initial interview: community, hospital, and nursing home. The hospital and nursing home subsamples were intended to be random samples in which an equal number of people would have an equal chance of becoming an MSSP or CSS participant. Randomness did not occur. Statistical analyses later showed that the more frail individuals were referred to MSSP. Because of this lack of randomness and consequent lack of representativeness, the CSS hospital and nursing home subsamples are excluded from our present analyses.

The CSS community sample, the subject of our analyses, is known as the "CID File Group" and is made up of individuals randomly selected from the Medi-Cal Central Identification (CID) File of all Medi-Cal eligibles. The relatively large size of this subsample (n = 1,303) allows extrapolation of our findings to the larger California Medi-Cal population. Analyses of the Medi-Cal expenditures of this "CID File Group" and those of a statewide random sample of five thousand elderly Medi-Cal recipients showed no statistically significant differences ($p. \leq 0.05$) in the average expenditures between the groups but variance of the CID group's Medi-Cal expenditures was significantly less than the variance of the five thousand group. From this we conclude that, on average, the "CID File Group" (i.e., the CSS for our present purposes) is comparable to the California statewide elderly Medi-Cal population. There are, however, some reservations about its general application to those Medi-Cal recipients with very high levels of expenditures.

No comparable data set on low-income elderly are available to determine definitively the national representativeness of our sample. However, at least along several dimensions the CSS sample is similar to the nation's poor elderly population (e.g., male-to-female sex ratio; predominance of spouseless white women; and mean age of about seventy-five). In these days of diminishing resources for social science survey research, we may never have a truly representative national longitudinal sample survey of low-income elderly. Decision makers may always have less than complete information on which to base policies.

Sample Formation

During the summer of 1980 we began forming the CSS. Administratively, the MSSP contracted with the California State University and Colleges System to establish the sampling sites' offices, hire and train interviewers, and actually carry out the interviews. Professor David L. Decker, Ph.D., from San Bernardino State College, was the southern coordinator and was responsible for the four southern locations:

Site	Number of CSS Respondents
• West Los Angeles	302
• East Lost Angles	86
• Long Beach	203
• San Diego	104
	695

Professor Anabel O. Pelham, Ph.D., from San Francisco State University, was the northern coordinator and was responsible for the four northern locations:

Site	Number of CSS Respondents
• Eureka	42
• San Francisco	238
• Oakland	287
• Santa Cruz	41
	608

The sampling locations were chosen purposely to be in the same areas as the MSSP experimental sites although the two staffs—MSSP and CSS—were completely different and kept separate.

Twenty-three CSS interviewers were hired full time. The staff was supplemented with occasional part-time help and translators. All interviewers were upper-division or graduate students or recent graduates from the CSUC system, most of whom had studied in the field of aging. All interviewers underwent several statewide training sessions to become familiar with the survey's objectives, the interview instrument, and data quality control procedures. Interviewers were paid a base salary plus travel expenses and a per-interview amount. Interviews were always face-to-face and usually done in respondents' homes. The actual participants in the survey received a fifteen dollar honorarium per interview. The total cost of each interview, excluding data processing costs, was approximately $170 per interview in fiscal year 1980–81 and about $210 per interview in fiscal year 1981–82.

The interviews used in these present analyses were carried out between August 1980 and June 1983. The initial interviews were completed in the first seventeen months. We have told the gritty day-by-day operation of the survey elsewhere and suggest that anyone who is to embark on survey research, particularly survey research with the poor elderly, look at our account (Pelham and Clark 1986a).

Survey Instrument

The CSS interview instrument is virtually the same as the MSSP questionnaire, which was based on an "anthology" of standard questions and indices used in long-term care practice and research. The major sections of the CSS interview instrument are:

- Demographics
- Activities of Daily Living (Katz 1963)
- Instrumental Activities of Daily Living (Lawton and Brody 1969)

- Short Portable Mental Status Questionnaire (Pfeiffer 1975)
- Life Satisfaction "Z" Scale (Adams 1969; Wood, Wylie, and Shaefor 1969)
- Family Characteristics
- Informal Support
- Social Service and Public Housing Use
- Acute and Chronic Conditions
- Health Status
- Medical-related Information

To insure the quality of the interview data, 240 inter-rater reliability interviews were carried out, encompassing more than 90 percent of the MSSP clinical staff and the CSS interviewers. On the functional sections dealing with specific indices, the statewide level of agreement was 93 percent, well above the accepted norm of 85 percent (Scherf 1982, 1983). James Lubben (1984) carried out an exhaustive account of the development of the MSSP and CSS instrument, with an abundance of psychometric data on the quality of specific items, and issues of reliability and validity.

Quantitative Methods

Interview data were combined with Medi-Cal and Medicare use and expenditure data and attrition information to form the CSS data sets. The proprietary statistical package used on the data was SAS ® ™. Marleen L. Clark carried out all the statistical analyses presented here. In addition to the standard descriptive statistics and multivariate regression procedures, we report on the results of an event history approach to the analysis of long-term care data. This analysis, the first of this type concerned with long-term care and designed by Leonard S. Miller and his associates (1984), is based on a dynamic modeling that predicts individuals' movements between care environments.

The basic building blocks of the model are individual movements between residency settings: community, acute hospital care, temporary nursing home, permanent nursing home care, dropout (i.e., voluntary attrition), and death. Time lines, or event histories, are constructed for all individuals, marking the dates when they entered and left institutional care, either hospital or nursing home, when they died, or when they dropped out for any reason (e.g., moved to another area). Figure 2–1 illustrates the six settings, more formally known as "states," and the direction of movements between them.

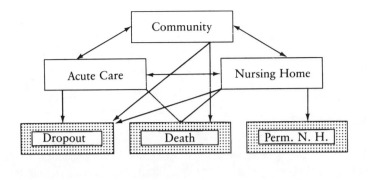

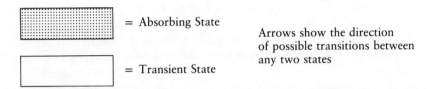

= Absorbing State

Arrows show the direction
of possible transitions between
any two states

= Transient State

Source: Multipurpose Senior Services Program: Impact Analysis, 1983–84, MSSP Evaluation
Unit, University of California, Berkeley, 1985.

Figure 2–1. Model of movements between residency settings

Transition rates—how "fast" or "slow" an individual moves between settings—are estimated and can be transformed into predictions of the number
of days the individual is expected to reside in each setting in a given time
period.

The utility of this approach to the analysis of long-term care can be sum-
marized in two words: dynamics and interdependence. Because the model
deals with movement, it is in contrast to static models, which rest on the
assumption that the system under study has reached some equilibrium. This
condition is rarely the case in social processes. And, the movements being
studied are not independent of each other (e.g., if you are in a hospital your
chances of entering a nursing home are much higher than if you are at home);
the modeling procedures used in these analyses permit examination of all
transition rates simultaneously.

Besides being able to estimate the experimental effect of MSSP, the event
history approach is useful for planning purposes. For example, given a low-
income elderly population with a certain set of characteristics (e.g., age, sex,
and functional status), what can we expect to be the annual use of nursing
home and hospital days? If no policy intervention is made to affect these use
patterns, what can we expect to be the public cost? Given that we can identify
the type of people most likely to use nursing home care and hospital care,

how can we communicate this information in a timely fashion to practitioners when they are at the point of accepting people as clients into their programs? These are the kinds of issues we discuss in chapter 12, "Planning and Policies."

Qualitative Methods

In addition to the quantitative results, we also use a qualitative research method from the field of ethnographic reporting. For particular topics we chose from among the respondents those individuals who were within the range of the modal characteristics of that topic. For example, in the next chapter we discuss the "modal" or typical respondent and present the stories of Judy Anderson and Iris Carlton (all names are fictitious). To arrive at specific individuals, we first determined the modal characteristics of several important variables (e.g., age, sex, and marital status) of the entire CSS sample. We then sorted all respondents according to specific criteria depending on the topic (e.g., being "old-old" or ethnicity) and identified those who met the criteria characteristics. For convenience we limited the respondents to those who lived in northern California. After verifying that they were still alive, we called them for interviews in the order they appeared on the printout. Only one of the thirteen individuals contacted for the vignette interviews refused. Anabel O. Pelham carried out all vignette interviews.

Frankly, we were surprised by the variety of stories our respondents told us about their lives and situations. The stories range from the lusty life of Judy Anderson, to the quiet, compliant, but independent Iris Carlton, to the exotic but difficult childhood of Rhea Majian, and the abject loneliness of Agnes Hughes. Although all share the common economic status of living in, at, or near poverty, their lives and histories are very different except for several characteristics. First, none was ever very wealthy and at best was in the lower middle class economic status throughout an entire life. What this means is that the best predictor of one's economic status after age sixty-five is one's status before age sixty-five. One's income certainly declines significantly when one becomes sixty-five but one does not suddenly become poor in old age. Spousal separation—divorce, legal separation, desertion, or death—causes more sudden and precipitous slides into poverty than does the aging process itself.

The second characteristic our vignette subjects share is the lack of a spouse, which is not surprising given their economic status. Interestingly, for those who had a spouse at one time, we usually heard a history of unsatisfactory married life. Given increased rates of divorce and separation in our present times, we are not sure what this will mean when the "baby boom" cohort reaches old age. If younger women do not gather assets while they can and/

or society does not allow them full access to the complete range of occupations with equal compensation schedules, it may mean significantly increased poverty rates in the next century and even greater numbers of poor women.

Philosophical Framework

Underlying our methodologies is a basic analytic framework that we should make explicit so that the reader may place our findings in a larger context. As chapter 11 points out in detail, the field of aging is the scene of jousting analytic frameworks—as perhaps befits a young field such as gerontology. The quest for a unified theory that explains and predicts the aging process, while connecting the phenomena to other fields, is an ongoing venture with no "right answer" in sight. For our own part, we advocate for an approach that incorporates both a macro-level analysis of the social and economic structures and man-made policies that influence the outcomes of life trajectories, and, at the micro level, analyses that examine how individuals perceive, interact, give meaning to, modify through an interpretative process, adapt to (or not), and change the phenomena of human aging. Underlying this macro and micro approach is a belief that reality is socially constructed. That is, humans are the ones who give meaning to and place value on phenomena— no *a priori* reality exists out there waiting to be revealed. Further, we believe that these meanings and values tend to reinforce the dominant social class and its economic interests.

In this book we concentrate on the micro level. The "unit of analysis" is the individual. A detailed analysis of the larger social and economic forces that influence the CSS participants is beyond our present level of resources. Ideally, this book would provide both macro and micro analyses, since we conceive these frameworks reflecting off one another like a hall of mirrors. As it is, we ask the reader to keep in mind this limitation and remember that a full understanding of poverty among the aged requires an analysis of the social and economic structures that permit over 3 million aged to live on less than $500 a month—for the rest of their lives.

For now we leave behind these major issues and turn to the actual participants in the CSS to listen to their stories and to discuss the major demographic characteristics of the respondents. We begin the next chapter with Judy Anderson and Iris Carlton, our "modal," or most typical, of the old and poor.

3
Demographics

Judy Anderson

Judy is a large woman with large features. Thin, pale red hair cut into a short pageboy style frames delicate, fair skin. She is dressed in stained synthetic fabric pants and print overblouse. She makes dolls to supplement her income.

Judy hunches over, elbows resting on knees. A European-style cigarette hangs between fingertips turned brown by sixty years of smoking. "And my doctor still says I'm in disgusting good health—even at seventy-five years young. I will live to ninety-nine and die. I know that because I'm somewhat psychic." She recalls several instances of prediction and clairvoyance. "I also had a psychic experience when I met my husband. I was a billing clerk for Westinghouse and living at the Polk Hotel in San Francisco. That was before the arsonist set fire to it. I survived the great Polk Hotel fire. One evening after work I was sitting at the bar drinking with friends, when a dark man walked in. I never look up at the customers or men that come in the door, but I did this time. Something like electricity went through me and I knew I would marry him."

Judy has been married four times and refers to each as "my husband," except for "the bigamist." Judy did have four husbands but learned later that the second, "or was it the third?", had abandoned a wife and four daughters to live with Judy on a two room houseboat in Seattle. The bigamist met a tragic end and Judy's recounting of this chapter in her life reveals much about her character. Dan had gone into town on business or errands and late in the afternoon Judy heard the clomp, clomp of unfamiliar shoes on the planks connecting the boat to the docks. A small woman and four young girls stood at the door. The stranger said she was Dan's wife and these were his children.

Judy had been cooking a beef stew all morning and made a mental note that there would be plenty to feed a large dinner group. Judy made peanut butter and jelly sandwiches for the girls and sent them out back to catch crawdads to feed the cat. She and the woman talked while she stirred the stew.

Judy then heard Dan's familiar step on the plank. He entered the room, paled, and took a seat at the table. Judy served up heaping bowls of stew. While they ate in silence she went into the other room and packed her husband's suitcase. She handed it to him and told him to go home to his family. She said she would simply claim him deceased in seven years—no questions asked. He and the chidren departed in the car. Night fell and Judy again was awakened by the sound of unfamiliar feet on her houseboat. She learned that Dan, the wife, and the four girls had been hit by a train when their car stalled on railroad tracks. She was asked to follow and identify the pitiful remains. How did the authorities know of her? Dan had carried her name and address on a note in his coat pocket.

Judy's life has been marked by a series of such tragic events. She had an unhappy childhood and spent most of her formative years in boarding schools and foster homes. Her mother was an accomplished dressmaker and seamstress who lived in Santa Cruz. Her mother also managed cottages (a motel) two blocks from where Judy now lives.

Judy's mother had wanted a son. Judy was told that her mother tried to send her back to the hospital when she was born. She was an only child and tried to be a boy for her mother but it did not work. "They did not have those sex-change operations in those days." Her mother beat her often and broke a broomstick over her back when she was late washing dishes.

Judy was born with amblyopia (lazy eye) and is partially blind. She can only see shapes and colors with the left eye but continues to sew very well.

Judy grew up without a father. He was caught molesting her when she was three and immediately divorced by her mother. She met him again at age thirteen and still did not like him. Judy was later raped by her mother's boyfriend and was packed off to another boarding school.

She spent some time with her mother's woman friend, who Judy later learned was a prostitute. Judy liked the woman but did not like sharing her bed when she had customers—which happened frequently. Judy lived for fifteen years in Fresno and learned the art and craft of dressmaking. Her attempts to work as an employee for her mother failed when her mother refused to pay her. Later, when Judy found jobs outside the home her mother took her paychecks except for bus fare and coins for coffee. While working, Judy compared notes with other girls and learned that they were paying their mothers only five dollars a week for room and board. Judy soon did the same and traded dates with merchants in exchange for cashing her paychecks.

"Five dollars was a lot of money then. I told Mother that the rest of the money was in my purse and that was where it was going to stay. She did not like it and tried to marry me off to every man that came over. One night she confronted my date and insisted on knowing his intentions. She embarrassed me so badly I would have sunk through a hole in the floor if it would open up."

Judy has worked as a waitress, office worker, and supervisor of an answering service. She was also the first female taxi driver in Santa Cruz. One of her favorite jobs was in a cabinet shop in San Francisco during World War II. She showed leadership qualities, signed up for the union, and was offered the position of supervisor at $1.50 an hour—twice the salary of the other women. The money was appreciated. Judy was now caring for her mother who was a patient at the University of California San Francisco Medical Center. Her mother died of cancer in 1943 at age fifty-three, leaving Judy with a half-brother and sister on her father's side, and an aunt. Judy is not emotionally close to those relatives, but is extremely proud of recently discovering evidence that she is a direct descendent of Sir Francis Drake.

While working at the cabinet shop Judy became quite skilled with power tools. Her biggest and proudest project was the single-handed construction of five thousand torpedo vents. "I made everything but the screens. I just could not figure out how to get those screens to fit and work. I still cannot figure out how those darn things work."

Cancer took the life of her fourth, last, and favorite husband, Larry. Clarence was his real name but Judy renamed him Larry. Judy is not her real name either. She was born Mabel in Bryn Mawr, outside of Seattle, Washington. She adopted the name Judy as a child. Larry, on the other hand, was christened shortly after that fateful electric meeting on a bar stool in San Francisco.

"I told the bartender I would buy that man a drink if he would sit by me. He was dark and I learned later he was one-eighth American Indian and a house painter. He came over but told me he would be poor company because he was suffering with his sinus condition. I went down the street to a pharmacist friend and had him make up some special ointment. Larry told me if the medicine worked he would take me to the Ice Follies and dinner the next day, Sunday. Well, it worked and I went to his apartment in the morning.

"His kitchen was tiny and down some dark steps. I slipped on a paper match and turned my ankle. Larry picked me up and we went ahead to the Ice Follies. By the end of the show my foot was hurting and too swollen to walk. The doorman and a passing sailor and Larry got me into a cab. We went to San Francisco General and waited five hours for an X-ray. The doctor said I had a very unusual break but that it would heal all right. I could not pay him so I said 'Thank you.' The doctor was so pleased and surprised that I thanked him."

After the Polk Hotel fire, Judy stayed at the Lankanshire and had dinner every night with Larry. One afternoon, on the corner of Fifth and Market streets, Larry suggested she get a permanent for her hair and in the same breath asked her to marry him. They were married fourteen years even though he was impotent. Judy never had children and Larry suggested she have other men—"Just come back home." She opted not to and remarks, "The last time I was intimate was thirty-five years ago and I do not miss it one bit. You know, the trouble with men is that they all try to get you to do things you do not want to do. I no longer drink either; it is a waste of time in my estimation."

Judy now lives in a remodeled motel four blocks from the beach in Santa Cruz. The cottages were built in 1939 and she shares what she calls her "dump" with her "Japanese bobtail" cat Sir Stubby Stubblefield, Stubby for short. He loves buttermilk and cottage cheese and is afraid of men.

Judy still drives a car but has a chore worker help with the housework. Judy survives on what she calls "Social Insecurity" and makes and sells dolls and doll clothing to earn extra money. Sales are slow and she usually goes hungry the last ten days of the month. "I'll feed the cat before I'll feed me." She is a chain smoker and coughs frequently. Her two-room motel-cottage with a tiny kitchen and bath is piled waist-high with computer magazines—she's taking a correspondence computer course and earning 70s scores—yarn balls, a television, dolls, paper bags, a card table (itself piled high), a recliner, a rocker, and a small organ.

Judy has her laundry neatly hung and drying in the bathroom. Dishes are neatly washed and drying in the kitchen.

She has recently worked as a foster grandparent for teens on probation. She earned the nickname "Huggin' Grandma." She is now trying to find a job caring for elders part time.

Working and standing will be difficult because Judy cannot stand for long. She has had five operations on her left hip and is on her third artificial hip. Judy is a tough customer. Eight years ago she fell and broke her wrist. She packed it in ice herself until the landlady could take her to the hospital. The fractures were so serious it was feared she would lose the use of her hand. Judy decided to force herself to type with the hand two hours a day—crying in pain all the while. Her therapy worked and she still has the use of a crooked left arm. "You know," she says, "most people give up too soon and too easily."

Judy sews baby dolls, clown dolls, Victorian ladies with hoop skirts, and crochet dogs. Bodies, faces, and outfits are hand-sewn and of exceptional quality. The nylon stocking dolls sell the most. She takes them to restaurants and sits them on the table while sipping coffee and sells them to customers for twenty dollars each.

Judy is always ready to sew. Multiple needles are pushed into the cushion of the rocker that butts up against the wall and will not rock.

She likes television for company. "It makes you feel like somebody's here. I'm not much of a mixer. I enjoy being by myself. When I'm alone, I'm in good company."

Judy is a Mormon and receives church visitors at least once a month.

She also has a list of visiting missionary teachers to call and check in with. She has to move her dolls to play the organ and still believes the theme from *The Third Man* is her favorite tune.

Iris Carlton

Iris Carlton is a gentle, compliant woman with a soft hint of a Southern accent. Her life has been neither a battleground for conflict nor a grand adventure. "You know, men have protected me all my life. First there was my father, then my five brothers, then my husband, Ray. He came from a big family too." Only two of her brothers are still living, both in the deep south of Louisiana and Mississippi.

Iris moves carefully across a very dim living room into a worn reclining chair. "The chair used to belong to my husband. It still works perfectly and only has one torn spot on the right arm." She has covered the tear with a terrycloth dish towel. "It's nobody's business but mine about the hole and I don't mind."

She is dressed in forever wrinkled synthetic pants and print overblouse, white socks, and soft shoes. On top of that she wears her husband's worn plaid cotton dressing gown with a white scarf tucked around the collar.

Iris Carlton looks softly at the world through pale blue eyes framed by uneven white hair. "I just gave myself a haircut with my husband's toilet scissors. I just pinched a strand with one hand and snipped with the scissors with the other."

Iris is blind in one eye. At her feet is her dog, Verdi (named after the composer) who is seventeen and totally blind. Verdi is a scrawny, long-legged, long-haired mixture. Verdi is quite decrepit but follows Iris everywhere. Iris has been invited to visit Sunday out of town for a day but hates to leave Verdi alone. She may call later and decline the invitation.

At seventy-seven years old, Iris Carlton enjoys relatively good health. "I only take one pill for high blood pressure, don't use salt, and vitamin pills is all."

Iris still has all her teeth, has never had surgery, and even has no stretch marks from the births of her three children . . . and is proud of it, too. Iris has one son and two daughters. Her son is fifty now and lives in Alabama. The daughters are forty-eight and thirty-six and live nearby in East Bay towns. Their families have produced eight grandchildren and four great-grandchildren.

One daughter is coming today. Iris may spend the weekend visiting the other. She enjoys watching the older children shoot pool in her daughter's home. She sees the "girls" often and the oldest calls every day.

Gifts of new and used clothing add a lot of joy to Iris' day. She has them coordinated in the closet and is most proud of a cranberry-colored woven wrap sweater. She also appreciates pants suits. "I even wear pants to church." Iris is not hard on clothes or shoes, either. She has had one pair of soft fabric shoes for ten years.

Gifts from her family are also a pleasure and surprise at Christmas time. The family draws names but Iris still receives a bounty, including a winter rain coat, sweater vests, bathrobes, night gowns, and perfumes.

Iris' son-in-law comes to vacuum the rugs and change light bulbs. He stops by on the way to work to run errands, do chores, and brings bags of dog food for Verdi.

Iris also enjoys the visits of church friends. They bring a lot of food. She has just gotten over a cold that kept her coughing for twenty-one days, during which time church friends would check in and bring food without disturbing her.

Iris is a devout Methodist. She had changed her religious affiliation when she married, to please her husband, but when he died she went back to her former faith.

Every Sunday at 9:45 A.M. a friend from church picks up Iris and drives her to church services. Iris plays the piano for services and pot luck gatherings, mostly hymns and sing-along tunes. She is attracted to the multiple nationalities and intergenerational elements in her church. (During the week the church is a day-care center.) The same multi-ethnic housing patterns are welcomed in her working-class neighborhood.

Iris lives in a pink painted four-plex. Her building and lawns are in need of repair, but she does not seem to notice. Iris knows the neighbor families and the children's names. She often meets them around the building's dumpster and mailboxes.

On her cork bulletin board on the kitchen wall are extra door keys for all the apartments pinned among physicians' businesses cards. She is the trusted gatekeeper for late children or those who need a spare key. Teen neighbors that she helped to raise often visit and talk over their problems.

Family, neighborhood, and church activities each occur almost daily and flow into a pattern of everyday life. Belonging to a church made an important difference during the years that Iris cared for her ill husband, Ray.

Iris met Ray in Mississippi. They attended high school together. She went to college to study the piano, and he did not go on. Music began for Iris when she fell off a horse and broke her arm. The fracture was serious and did not heal straight. Fearing the loss of the use of her arm, Iris, at age seven, began piano lessons. She soon played for the Methodists and Baptists and community socials. If there is any passion in Iris' life it is for the piano. When she plays she leans into the keyboard with her body and a faraway look covers her face.

Iris was born in Greensberg on the Green River in Green County, Kentucky. She lived there until she was twelve and in the eighth grade. Her father was a partner in a barrel-making company. He decided to buy a share-cropping plantation of sixteen thousand acres and moved the family to Crowder, Mississippi.

The plantation workers were black and Iris was taught not to be prejudiced. To this day she appreciates multi-ethnic diversity.

Iris married Ray in Mississippi before making a planned move west. "My family insisted we get married before going to California. Ray wanted to get going but there was my father and my five brothers to deal with. We lived in Los Angeles for a year and Ray built the County Hospital. He made good money there. Then we moved to Oakland. Ray worked as a machinist for the H. J. Heinz Catsup Company—and he never did get his hands dirty."

Iris has never occupied a salaried position. Her husband did not approve of her working outside the home. Iris took baby-sitting jobs and earned as much as five dollars a session.

Serious illness entered Ray's life in the form of tuberculosis. The doctors collapsed his lung to stop the spread of the infection. Ray's breathing problems worsened during the next ten years. He developed lung cancer. Iris remembers that he had only smoked for a while and then stopped. Ray's collapsed lung and part of the other was removed. He was left with about one-fourth of a seriously compromised respiration system.

Apparently the earlier diagnosis of tuberculosis had been an error—no evidence of it was found. The purposeful collapse of the lung had been an error.

Iris spent a lot of time in hospitals during this period but "always went to Sunday church."

Soon Ray was put on a home respirator and his long downhill struggle began. Iris cared for him at home until his death and feels like the state of California was good to them in covering costs towards the end.

Iris understands about the wrong diagnosis and knows the radical surgical intervention that collapsed Ray's probably healthy lung most likely was unnecessary. She further realizes that the respiratory stress created by the deficit probably contributed to the lung cancer and her husband's painful death. Yet these facts rest as lightly on Iris' spirit as her fingers on the keyboard of her piano. She has accepted what she cannot alter.

Iris has lived in Oakland all her adult life. Her apartment has been home for the past thirteen years, and is subsidized so that out-of-pocket costs for rent are $179.50 a month [1985]. She also pays $2.50 month for floodlight protection and $6.50 to the apartment manager for garbage collection costs.

Iris' apartment is clean and spacious. She enjoys a picture window in the living room that sheds light on a hanging multisided silver bell and throws rainbow colors in the afternoon. Her bath, bedroom, and kitchen are tidy and things kept in a predictable place for Verdi's convenience.

Iris has collected afghans for the sofas, family pictures, knickknacks, and tiny tea cups and saucers. One of her two reclining chairs faces the television and Reader's Digest hardback books line the shelves.

Iris plays the piano daily and listens to the five and six o'clock news on the radio. "I guess President Reagan is doing the best he can but I am worried about Social Security and all the people being murdered you hear about on the news."

Old television shows fill part of her day. She usually watches two or three while doing housework. "It takes me twice as long to do anything, but I enjoy every minute of every day. If I get blue I just get busy cleaning house. I stay busy all day long with just little jobs."

Washing clothes has gotten a lot easier since her chidren surprised her with a new washer hooked up conveniently in her kitchen.

Reading religious books is another important part of Iris' day. A neighbor woman gave her a hand-held plastic magnifying glass. Iris also listens faithfully to the radio from 7:00 to 8:30 P.M. for the Bible reading program.

Iris is able to manage financially on Social Security and an additional monthly check from Supplemental Security Income and the State Supplemental Payment program. She owes no money and has never charged anything. She and Ray always saved for purchases. Her son has asked Iris for years to move south and live with his family and have more security. She declines in favor of independence—"Besides, I hate the heat."

Iris is really quite independent. She takes the bus everywhere on a four-dollar monthly senior "Fast Pass." She talks and listens to lonely riders talk about life's problems and potentials. She feels she can do some good just riding the bus and listening.

"No one has ever been unkind to me," Iris says. "All people are helpful— but I am careful with my purse."

Who Are the Old and Poor?

The most direct answer to the question, "Who are the old and poor?" lies in the stories of our two vignettes. The old and poor are white women in their mid-seventies living alone in rented apartments or houses, with some chronic functional limitations. Although Judy did not have children, this is atypical. Most poor elderly—of both genders—have children who remain in frequent contact, as do Iris'. As we see from these two stories, and the ones that follow, these people are active and productive, from making and selling dolls to riding the bus and listening to lonely riders.

What impressed us about these two women is how different they are, given that they are "modal" respondents. The somewhat eccentric and exotic Judy and the more compliant Iris represent, in a statistical sense, typical poor elderly, yet it is hard to imagine two more different personalities. Although we did not plan it this way, the juxtaposition of the two "typical" elderly underscores how heterogeneous are the elderly, even when they share major socioeconomic traits. We should all keep this in mind as we discuss statistical findings and trends.

The stories also support the notion that personality acts as a constant throughout one's history. Judy's and Iris' life stories, abbreviated as they are, suggest that their respective sets of distinguishing behavioral and emotional characteristics, developed early in life, continue more or less the same into old age.

From these very personal stories we now examine some of the quantitative data that adds up all of the Judys and Irises to give a concise—if somewhat dry—portrait of the old and poor.

Aggregate United States Statistical Data

In 1986, nearly 3.5 million people sixty-five and over lived below the poverty line. This represents a poverty rate among the eldery of 12.4 percent, or about one out of every eight elderly. This rate is dramatically less than the 1959 35.2 percent poverty rate. No doubt Social Security cost-of-living adjustments (COLAs), in place since 1970, were instrumental in creating this twenty-five year decline in poverty rates among the elderly. However, the 1984 rate for people sixty-five and over living below 125 percent of the poverty line—the "near poor"—was 21.2 percent, meaning an additional 2.3 million elderly people are marginally poor (U.S. Bureau of the Census 1985c).

The 1985 poverty line was $5,156 a year for an elderly person living alone and $6,503 a year for an elderly couple, or $430 and $542 a month respectively.

U.S. Census data show that although white women make up the greatest number of poor aged—two of every three poor elderly people are women—the poverty rates are much greater among minorities. For example, older blacks are nearly three times as likely to be poor as older whites (31.7 percent versus 10.7 percent). Poverty among elderly Hispanics is about two times the rate for aged whites (21.5 percent versus 10.7 percent). The poverty rates for aged blacks who are female heads of households is shocking: 60.5 percent.

The chief reason women are more likely to be poor in old age than are men is that women are more likely to be poor when they are younger. Despite changes in the economy and hefty antidiscrimination legislation, this pattern is not likely to change. Victor Fuchs' study of the economic well-being of women twenty-five to sixty-four, compared with that of men, concluded that it did not improve between 1959 and 1983 and, in fact, decreased (Fuchs

1986). The insidious consequences of a lifetime of occupational segregation and lower wage rates, along with marital separation, are compounded for those women who did not participate in the work force because of marriage and family rearing and then, at widowhood, suffered a reduction in their spouse's Social Security benefit of about one-third (Warlick 1985). For about 20 percent of the widows, who are, on average, about fifty-five years old at widowhood, the death of a spouse is tantamount to receiving a life sentence—about twenty years—of impoverishment (U.S. Bureau of the Census 1985b).

Although the U.S. Census data provide us with some of the primary characteristics of the aged poor, we still do not know very much about their detailed demographic data, their family life, their physical functioning, their use of social and medical services, or other areas of interest. To better understand their general condition we turn to specific data of the California Senior Survey (table 3–1).

Gender

Gender distribution shows a prominance of women among the aged poor, a full 70 percent, whereas the general elderly population is made up of about 60 percent women. The sex ratio shows about four men for every ten women, much less than the current ratio for the elderly, in general, which is about two men for every three women (Myers 1985). These differences become more exaggerated among the older groups, and in the eighty-five-and-older group the ratio is less than one man for every three women.

Age

The age distribution in table 3–1 shows that the aged poor are much older than the general elderly population. For example, the general U.S. elderly population has about 61 percent in age bracket sixty-five to seventy-four, but the CSS group has only 41 percent. Similarly, the CSS group has about 21 percent in the eighty-five-and-older group, but the U.S. elderly population has only 9 percent. This eighty-five-and-older group is the fastest-growing age group within the elderly population and we discuss this group and its special problems in chapter 10. However, although this group is growing rapidly, it still will not comprise over 20 percent of the general elderly population until some time between the years 2025 and 2050 (Myers 1985). In a sense, this CSS subgroup provides us a preview of the kinds of societal problems associated with having a sizeable, very aged subpopulation.

The actual average age of the CSS respondents, 75.2 for males and 77.1 for females, means that they can expect from eight to nine more years of life. These figures are from life expectancy data for the general elderly population

Table 3–1
Characteristics of the respondents of the California Senior Survey at the initial interview

Characteristic	Male n 425	Male % 29.6	Female n 1012	Female % 70.4	Total n 1437	Total % 100.0
Age:						
65–74	202	47.5	387	38.3	589	41.0
75–84	153	36.0	395	39.0	548	38.1
85+	70	16.5	230	22.7	300	20.9
Average Age	75.2		77.1		76.5	
Standard Deviation	6.8		7.8		7.6	
Ethnic/Racial:						
White	235	55.3	614	60.7	849	59.1
Black	71	16.7	168	16.6	239	16.6
Hispanic	32	7.5	97	9.6	129	9.0
Asian	37	8.7	69	6.8	106	7.4
Other	50	11.8	64	6.3	114	7.9
Marital Status:						
Married	205	48.4	150	14.8	355	24.7
Widowed	99	23.4	667	65.9	766	53.3
Divorced/Separated	75	17.6	150	14.8	225	15.7
Single	43	10.1	43	4.3	86	6.0
Other	2	0.5	2	0.2	4	0.3
Living Arrangement:						
Alone	156	36.8	543	53.9	699	48.8
With spouse	130	30.6	110	10.9	240	16.9
With spouse & children	39	9.2	15	1.5	54	3.7
With children only	16	3.8	107	10.6	123	8.7
With brother or sister	5	1.2	24	2.4	29	2.0
With other family	19	4.5	79	7.8	98	6.8
Board & care	15	3.5	20	2.0	35	2.4
Other	44	10.4	110	10.9	154	10.7
Average Number of Living Children:						
(for those with children: 73.3%)	3.4		2.9		3.1	
Standard Deviation	2.5		2.1		2.2	
Average Number of Living Grandchildren:						
(for those w/grandchildren: 69.0%)	8.9		8.5		8.6	
Standard Deviation	9.7		8.5		8.8	
Educational Level:						
None	28	6.6	86	8.5	114	7.9
Grade school	184	43.3	430	42.6	614	42.8
High school	119	28.0	346	34.2	465	32.4
High school+	94	22.1	149	14.7	243	16.9
Average Years of Education:						
Standard Deviation	8.4		7.9		8.1	
	4.0		4.0		4.0	
Mental Status:						
Intact	369	86.7	830	82.0	1199	83.4
Mild	42	9.9	124	12.3	166	11.6
Moderate	12	2.9	48	4.7	60	4.1
Severe	2	<1.0	10	1.0	12	<1.0

(continued)

Table 3–1 (*continued*)

Characteristic	Male n 425	Male % 29.6	Female n 1012	Female % 1437	Total n 70.4	Total % 100.0
Number of ADL Dependencies:						
0 (Independent)	361	85.0	822	81.3	1183	82.8
1–2	45	10.6	145	14.3	190	13.2
3–4	16	3.6	29	2.8	45	3.2
5–6 (Dependent)	3	0.8	16	1.6	19	1.3
Number of IADL Dependencies:						
0 (Independent)	30	7.0	43	4.2	73	5.1
1–2	231	54.5	533	52.7	764	53.1
3–4	83	19.6	233	23.0	316	22.0
5–6	56	13.0	129	12.8	185	12.9
7–8 (Dependent)	25	5.9	74	7.3	99	6.9
Self-Reported Health Status:						
Good	176	41.6	383	38.3	559	39.3
Fair	188	44.4	458	45.8	646	45.4
Poor	59	14.0	159	15.9	218	15.3
Average Number of Chronic Conditions:						
(Out of 25 possible conditions)	2.2		2.8		2.6	
Standard Deviation	1.8		2.0		1.9	

(Shanas and Maddox 1985). Alma McMillan and her associates from the Health Care Financing Administration (1983) have shown that the aged poor under eighty apparently experience higher mortality rates than the nonpoor, so the eight to nine more years of life should be interpreted more as maxima than as averages.

Race and Ethnicity

The ethnic and racial data in table 3–1 reveal one of the larger differences between the general elderly and the poor elderly. For the United States as a whole, about 90 percent of the elderly are white, 8 percent black, and 2 percent other racial or ethnic groupings. In contrast to this 10 percent of nonwhite population, the CSS contains almost 40 percent nonwhite. This proportion is even greater than the U.S. Census data for those below the poverty line, which indicates that nonwhites make up 23 percent of the poor elderly. The representation of a greater share of nonwhites in the CSS group is explained by California's more diverse racial composition and our purposeful sampling strategy. This strategy included one site that was almost entirely Hispanic (East Los Angeles) and another (San Francisco) that contains the highest number of legal immigrants per capita of any city in the United States. This higher proportion of nonwhites allows us to treat at length the question of ethnicity among the elderly in chapter 7.

Marital Status

The marital status patterns of the poor elderly are similar to those of the general elderly but the trends are more exaggerated among the poor. For example, for the general elderly population in 1984, men were twice as likely to be married as older women (AARP 1985). For our CSS participants, men were three times as likely to be married. Similarly, half of all older women in 1984 were widows, but two-thirds of the CSS women were widows.

Among the poor, the proportion of those divorced increased only one or two percentage points in the last ten years (Tissue 1978), but for all older persons, the number of divorced individuals increased over three times as fast in the preceding twenty years. Although divorced older people presently represent only 4 percent of all older persons, we can expect this group to increase significantly in the coming years, given the divorce rate among the younger population.

These larger societal trends may create more spouseless individuals among the elderly in the future but presently, most of the general elderly are married (52 percent). However, most of the poor elderly are spouseless and, as we saw from Judy's and Iris' stories, spouselessness can have both positive and negative dimensions. We explore different aspects of this in Chapter 4, about the family, and in chapter 8, about widows.

Living Arrangement

Most CSS respondent live alone, which is in contrast to the general elderly population, about 30 percent of whom live by themselves. This living arrangement is consistent with the marital status patterns of the two groups. What is similar between the two groups is that there seems to be a preference of *not* living with their children. Chapter 4 discusses this preference, termed "intimacy at a distance," which apparently exists in most industrial societies. The living arrangement preference seems to have emerged even though almost three-quarters of the CSS respondents have an average of three children and are part of a three-generation family with an abundance of grandchildren.

Educational Level

On average, CSS respondents have completed grade school. Minor differences appear to exist between genders, but the CSS educational attainment level is about three years less than the elderly population as a whole. A more detailed analysis in chapter 7 reveals significant differences among racial and ethnic groupings. We find there that a large percentage of Asian and Hispanic women have had no schooling, which means they are most likely illiterate in their first language as well as in English. Programs that attempt to serve these minority women will have to use media other than print—even literature in the native language—to make known available services.

Mental Status

The levels of intellectual impairment are determined through use of the Short Portable Mental Status Questionnaire (SPMSQ) developed by Eric Pfeiffer (1975). The questionnaire contains ten questions asked of the respondents, such as "What is today's date?" "Who is the president?" "Please count backward from twenty, subtracting three each time." The score is adjusted by race and education and up to two errors is considered "normal." The questionnaire focuses on organic brain deficit and is not meant as a diagnostic tool for identifying psychological impairments such as depression. As such, the questionnaire provides a measure of cognitive impairment. The CSS data reveal that relatively few respondents are less than "intact."

No comparable data exist at the national level for the noninstitutionalized population, but smaller sample surveys also reveal few noninstitutionalized elderly with less than an intact score. Although this pattern seems to hold for the noninstitutionalized elderly, regardless of income levels, surveys of nursing home patients show a completely different pattern. Here, chronic and significant cognitive impairment is estimated for 56 percent of residents (National Center for Health Statistics 1979; Federal Council on the Aging 1981). Perhaps more than any other single characteristic, cognitive impairment separates the noninstitutionalized elderly from the nursing home residents.

Functional Disabilities: Activities of Daily Living and Instrumental Activities

A consensus seems to be emerging in the field of gerontology that accepts the definition of health among the elderly as one based on level of functioning, a position first proferred by the World Health Organization in 1959 (Shanas and Maddox 1985). To measure the levels of functioning ability, two indexes are becoming increasingly accepted as the instruments of choice among researchers and practitioners. They are the Activities of Daily Living (ADL), developed by Sidney Katz and his associates (1963, 1970), and the Instrumental Activities of Daily Living (IADL), developed by M. Powell Lawton and Elaine Brody (1969, 1972). The ADL is a six-item index that measures the more basic and personal tasks such as eating, bathing, and transfer (i.e., movement out of a bed into a chair and vice versa). The IADL, an eight-item index, measures functional ability in the areas of household management such as shopping, meal preparation, and telephoning. Both indexes are based on self-report of the respondent and both ask whether the person *does actually perform* the task, rather than asking if the person *could perform* the task. Also, both indexes define dependency based on whether the respondent receives assistance from another person in carrying out the task. If the person carries out the task with the aid of some assistive device, the person is deemed independent.

Data in table 3–1 reveal a pattern that seems to be consistent with other sample surveys: the elderly are generally able to carry out all the ADL tasks, but a much larger group needs assistance with one or more of the IADL tasks (Shanas 1977; Tissue 1978). For example, the most recent national survey data indicate that 88 percent of all noninstitutionalized elderly are completely independent in all ADL tasks. This level of independence does change, however, from age group to age group. The sixty-five-to-seventy-four age group is 93.1 percent independent, but the eighty-five-and-older group is only 56.4 percent (Committee on an Aging Society 1985).

Other studies of disability levels, using other measures (and including all income levels), found that low-income groups have a much higher share of disability than do their more affluent peers. Lewis Butler and Paul Newacheck (1981) conclude that low income leads to lower levels of nutrition, housing, health care, and other necessities, and therefore to a greater likelihood that a chronic health condition will develop or worsen among the low-income groups.

Chapter 5 is devoted to an analysis of the functional levels of the poor elderly and what differences are attributable to age, gender, and ethnicity, as well as how functional status changes over time.

Self-Reported Health Status and Chronic Conditions

The self-reported health status data in table 3–1 do not reveal much difference between genders but are significant when compared to the general elderly population. In 1981, only 30.1 percent of the U.S. population sixty-five years old and older reported a health status of "fair or poor," compared to the poor elderly's 60.7 percent (National Center for Health Statistics 1984). The rates for the middle-aged (forty-five to sixty-four years) and for the young adults (seventeen to forty-four years) are 20 percent and 8.3 percent, respectively. This indicates that not only are the poor elderly in much worse health than the younger groups, but also that the prevalance of poor-health status is twice that of the elderly in higher-income groups.

The effects of income can also be seen in the number of chronic conditions reported by the CSS respondents. The CSS average is 2.6; the national average for the elderly is 1. The most common conditions are arthritis and high blood pressure.

Summary

After reviewing all these characteristics and keeping in mind the stories of Judy and Iris, a fairly complete outline emerges about who the old and poor are and their similarities and differences from the elderly in higher-income groups. The similarities are that the "typical" individual in both groups is a white woman who is spouseless, primarily due to widowhood. The women in both groups have children and are part of a three-generational family, although they tend to live alone.

The differences are, most notably, lesser income, which seems to be the result of a lifetime of living at or near poverty rather than a sudden shift of income status; lower levels of functional independence; and a higher incidence of chronic health problems. So, this group is not only poorer, but also sicker. Although we did not measure the adequacy of their housing, it is safe to assume the poor elderly's shelter is of lesser quality and in less safe neighborhoods than that of their more affluent counterparts.

Although the poor elderly have fewer resources (e.g., money, functional status, and health) than do the elderly in higher-income groups, they seem to be similar in another important area of their lives—the whole dimension of the family, its structure and interaction of its members. Our next chapter examines this area in detail.

4

The Family

Gertrude Aston

At ninety years old, Gertrude Aston is tiny, somewhat frail and slightly bent over. She moves slowly and is slightly unsteady from her fingertips to her slipper-covered feet. Her short, silver hair frames blue eyes that are usually serious but sparkle now and then at a distant recollection. Her rose dressing gown matches pink eyeglasses that appear almost too large for her face. She has one daughter and three granddaughters.

Gertrude was a "baby nurse," which shaped the nature of her life. She started private-duty nursing in homes in Germany. Before that she worked around her own home to help her mother and later worked as a housekeeper in her birthplace, Hamburg, Germany.

Although Gertrude trained as a baby nurse she never earned a license or degree. She maintains a thick German accent that becomes more understandable the longer she speaks. Gertrude's memory for specific words and details fails occasionally and she cannot remember the German words for "baby" or "child's nurse." No matter, she does not mind that she cannot remember; maybe she will think of it later.

Gertrude has lived for eight years in a small, one-room apartment with a kitchen in a high-rise senior housing complex behind Laguna Honda Hospital in San Francisco. The building is constructed of textured grey concrete and built into the side of a treeshaded hillside. Interior floors and walls are worn but not dirty. Door buzzers to the building have been broken for so long that an "informed entry" system is evolving among the tenants for security purposes. Gertrude's room is clean, dimly lit, and furnished with a single unmade bed and a small dining table in the center of her room. Lining her walls are little wood tables, a dresser, and a single large window. Photographs of family and her babies rest on every surface—the "babies" are actually young men and women on holidays and middle-aged adults posing with birthday gifts and at family gatherings. Many of these individuals, having reached adulthood, keep in contact with Gertrude and remain forever her babies.

Early family life in Hamburg found Gertrude the middle child in a family of three other sisters and brothers. All are dead now except for eighty-eight-year-old Bertha, who lives in Hamburg. Gertrude and Bertha visit over the telephone about once a month, more often if "something important" develops.

Gertrude Aston joined her brother in the United States in 1923. There was not an overwhelming compelling reason for immigrating to America. Gertrude does not remember suffering in Germany. "I don't care for politics and just follow suit with what the government wants." She arrived by ship to New York City and took the train to her brother's in San Francisco.

Gertrude lived with her brother and his wife and worked as a domestic until her brother's wife became acutely ill and died. "He was left alone and adrift with no children. He started seeing a Mexican woman who wanted to take over. He married her and she wanted to go to El Salvador. He moved there and built a beautiful estate. It all must have been too much for him, as he died three years later."

It was while attending a German social club in San Francisco that Gertrude Aston met the man who would become her husband. To this day Gertrude believes the union was an unfortunate choice. "He was an orphan and a seaman and he and his friends were rough. He came home always empty [without money]. We were married four years and I never saw him." Gertrude divorced him while he was at sea. "He never helped me or the child. He was a woman chaser. He even came to my house later trying to borrow money. I told him if he found any to bring me some because I need money, too."

After Gertrude's divorce she found herself quite alone in a still-alien country with a young daughter to support.

"I lived on Union Street at the time [now a posh street of boutiques and trendy restaurants]. I rented out the three front rooms and placed screens and barriers between the kitchen area and back rooms where Marge and I lived. A woman, living alone, can't be too careful."

Gertrude's tenants were mostly male and stayed in her home for long periods.

"I once had a tenant that was in the food business—I cannot remember his name—but one night he placed a large bag by the kitchen counter. At first I was frightened because he was not supposed to be in that part of the house. Marge and I peeked into the bag and found it full of groceries! Every week after that he left a bag of groceries. He told me it was extra from his business and that I should accept what fate provided. Marge thought of him as Santa Claus. He lived with me for many years and never failed to bring a bag of groceries every week."

Sometime later—Gertrude cannot remember when—she found a family that needed child care. The husband and wife were both physicians and were very supportive of Gertrude. She grew to care for them both. This extended family became so close that when the couple planned to move out of the area they invited Gertrude and Marge to relocate, too. Gerturde remembers struggling over the decision for a long time and then deciding to stay in San Francisco. As a going-away gesture, the wife attended to Gertrude's future employment by placing her name with a respected OB-GYN physician as a trusted baby nurse. Gertrude remembers, "I was never alone after that." The physician's secretary referred new mothers in need of child care to Gertrude and she remembers seeing a little gold star by her name on the secretary's list of mother's helpers.

Gertrude had other marriage offers in youth and middle age, but never remarried or felt like she had close men friends. "I had no time for a good time outside but I was never lonely. I had good jobs in good homes. I always worked for fine people. One year I joined my employers in Italy and lived for a year in Milano. When my employer families would travel I would travel, too."

Although Gertrude was employed she never felt financially secure. "The work was never paid the right price. It always kept me in the dark about if I had enough money."

Today, Gertrude's income is adequate to meet her needs, which are minimal, and she is immersed in a small, but close and caring, family. Marge and her husband live just over the hill and her twin granddaughters are now twenty-five years old and are in frequent contact. Marge calls three times a day to check in. The third granddaughter, who lives in Louisiana, calls every Sunday. Gertrude is very close to her twin granddaughters and helped to raise them.

"For a time I lived with Marge and cared for the twins. I would tuck them into bed for the evening and then go to my room. One night I found one of the twins asleep on the floor curled up in a ball outside my closed door. She had crawled out of her bed and tried to come to me. She could not reach the doorknob so she fell asleep. She was only fourteen months at the time! This happened three more times. I would awake and find little baby bundles outside my door!"

In addition to checking in three times a day, Gertrude's daughter helps with the shopping, carries in the bags, and puts away groceries. She regularly takes Gertrude out for rides "to see the sights." Every weekend Marge prepares a family dinner and brings Gertrude over, or sometimes the entire family goes out to dinner.

Friends and family members who own automobiles take Gertrude anywhere she wishes to go. Her daughter usually drives her to the doctor's office for a monthly checkup. Gertrude describes her physician, who is in his sixties, as a "wonderful, intelligent, very friendly man who always explains why."

While reporting on her physician, Gertrude becomes very serious and explains how much she depends upon Medicare. "In common I am healthy, but I take heart pills and water pills. I cannot eat salt."

Gertrude remembers a day last year when she became ill on the bus. "I could not breathe well and finally got myself home. The breathlessness lasted all day and during the evening I went to the manager and asked for oxygen. An ambulance came and they took me to French Hospital. I was there two weeks. I had water in my lungs. I take medication for it now and go to the doctor once a month for a checkup."

Gertrude has a good friend, Mrs Smythe, who lives in the same building. Mrs. Smythe immigrated from England and helps with paperwork, messages, and the telephone. Gertrude and Mrs. Smythe met in the elevator and the relationship got off to a problematic start, with each taking turns at ignoring the other. Today Gertrude and her friend frequent Pier 39, a tourist area of shops and restaurants on the Embarcadero in San Francisco, and sit in the sunshine and people-watch. On quieter days Gertrude sits in the building's garden. Mrs. Smythe has a reputation as a "character" in the building and is not well liked. Gertrude says that makes their friendship all the more special.

Gertrude Aston believes that the high point of her life occurred about twenty years ago when she won an opportunity to visit her family in Germany. She remembers clearly that her granddaughter was four years old at the time. It began with a trip Gertrude took to Reno, Nevada with a German secretary friend who worked for the Zellerbach Company. Gertrude was fooling around and won forty-two dollars on the nickel slot machines. She decided to play ten dollars worth of nickels on the dollar slot machines. She won five dollars. She played those and won a bell ringing a thousand dollars—a jackpot on the first try.

Gertrude spent the money on a freighter trip to Germany. She treasured the reunion with her family and her only sorrow was the death of her brother two weeks before her arrival.

Today Gertrude is a quiet, fragile, soft-spoken woman who spends most of her time in her tiny apartment. An In-Home Supportive Services worker from the county Department of Social Services comes in five days a week to clean. Every day, promptly at 2:45 P.M., the phone rings with Marge checking in. Channels to the outside are well-traversed by family and a friend.

Today, involvement in the rest of the world through television, radio, and books is relatively limited. Gertrude "was Lutheran" but never joined a church. Her daughter and grandchildren attend but Gertrude finds the city fog often too cold for outdoor travel to worship.

Gertrude recently fell from her bed and injured a knee. Bruises and soreness are gone but the shock and fear of another fall remains. Falling from the bed is a secret Gertrude keeps from her daughter. She worries that Marge will move her into her home. Such a fate could strain a fragile independence and a helping, loving relationship with breathing space for everyone. Gertrude believes that "when you are down in the dumps and have done right and been patient, you don't die. You get a little of the good side." This is really all Gertrude is wishing for now—a little on the good side for the remainder of her life.

Family Structure and Family Resources: Survey Results

Introduction

Gertrude Aston's story illustrates what more than four decades of survey research consistently reports: families actively and freely care for their elder members. Gertrude also personifies the elderly involved in the "stuff" of families: caring, loving, listening, mediating, approving, and acknowledging. She, like most of her cohorts, belongs to a multigenerational family, both receiving and giving assistance. What Gertrude's story highlights, not captured by our survey data, is the dynamic nature of the relationships. That is, when Gertrude was younger she gave more help and assistance than she received; now, she receives more.

Generally, however, the low-income elder's intergenerational interactions do not differ from the more affluent elderly. What does characterize the low-income elderly, in terms of family structure, is spouselessness and living alone. We begin our description of the CSS data by looking at these characteristics. After describing the family structure and types of family interaction we carry out multivariate analyses that explain and predict why some elders have more contact with their children than do others, and why some receive more help from their family and friends than do others. We end this chapter with some thoughts on the policy ramifications of our findings.

Family Structure

Number of Generations. Just as the elderly in general belong to multigenerational families, so do the low-income elderly. Ethel Shanas (1977) reports that 76 percent of her national probability sample are part of three- and four-generation families. We also found this true, in general, for the low-income elderly in California. We did find, however, that significant differences exist between ethnic/racial groupings and by gender (table 4–1). For example, Hispanic and Asian men and women are much more likely to belong to three-

Table 4–1

Percentage distribution of the number of generations, by ethnic/racial group and by gender

| | Ethnic/Racial Groups[a] | | | | | | | |
| Number of Generations | White | | Black | | Hispanic | | Asian[b] | |
	Male (n=235)	Female (n=614)	Male (n=71)	Female (n=168)	Male (n=32)	Female (n=97)	Male (n=37)	Female (n=69
1	36	23	45	37	19	18	16	4
2	11	10	6	10	3	7	3	4
3+	53	67	49	52	78	75	81	92

[a]Other groupings, such as American Indian and Filipinos, were excluded because of small cell sizes.
[b]"Asian" includes Chinese, Japanese, and Korean.

and four-generational families than whites and blacks. A startling finding is that a full 45 percent of the black men belong to only one-generation families.

The black group has a less extensive family, defined by blood relatives and by marriage, than one might imagine. No doubt the notoriously high black infant mortality rates influenced the present family composition. Prenatal care and birthing conditions, bad as they are now, were worse during the twenties and thirties, the childbearing years of the CSS respondents. Additionally, black men suffer relatively higher rates of hypertension and many die in their fourth and fifth decade. On the other hand, blacks may make up for this with what Donald Ball (1972) calls "fictive kin" (people unrelated by blood or marriage but who act like and who are treated like family members). However, the low-income black men may represent an "at risk" group because of an apparent lack of available family resources to draw upon during time of need.

Hispanic and Asian groups overwhelmingly belong to three-generation families or more. In fact, although not shown in table 4–1, not one Hispanic or Asian reported being "kinless" (i.e., without spouse, sibling, or child). Admittedly, this may be because most elderly Hispanics and Asians were probably brought to California by family members and their "kinless" peers never emigrated. Nonetheless, we are unlikely to find many true isolates among low-income elderly Hispanics and Asians.

Marital Status. More than any sociodemographic characteristic other than level of available economic resources, marital status distinguishes the poor elderly from the general elderly. Most poor elderly are spouseless. In contrast, for the United States as a whole, 1980 census data reveal that, for most elderly, spouses living together as a pair is the norm. This is particularly true for men; they are twice as likely to be married after sixty-four than are women. Women, on the other hand, are most likely to be widows. For the United States in 1980, 51 percent of women sixty-five and over were widows, while for men this percentage was only 14 percent (U.S. Bureau of the Census 1983). In addition, widowers have remarriage rates seven times higher than widows (U.S. Bureau of the Census 1983). After age seventy-five, the percentage of widowed women rises to 68 percent. For men it is still about three times less at 24 percent. Even though by age sixty-five about 94 percent of all women have been married at least once, death, divorce, and desertion have left about 62 percent of all women spouseless (U.S. Congress 1982). Spouseless women make up most of the U.S. elderly seventy-five and over.

Our own data show the predominance of spouseless women among the low-income elderly (displayed in chapter 7, table 7–2). This is true irrespective of ethnic grouping. Differences that do appear are found in the marriage rate of men in the different groupings. For example, 72 percent of the Hispanic men and 76 percent of the Asian men are married. These rates are in contrast to 42 percent of the white men and 33 percent of the black men.

Thomas Tissue (1978) also found this to be true in Social Security Administration's national sample of welfare recipients. Among these aged welfare recipients, men are three times as likely to be married as women. In fact, spouseless women make up 59 percent of that total, nationally representative sample. In our own California sample they represent about 62 percent of the total.

Living Arrangement. This follows marital status patterns. For the United States, five-sixths of the men live in a family setting, while only three-fifths of the women do. According to U.S. Census data, of the 7 million elderly people living alone in 1982 (about 30 percent of the total elderly population), most were women. Of those seventy-five years old and older, half of the women and about a fifth of the men lived alone (U.S. Bureau of the Census 1983b).

Our own data show a predominance of living alone among the white and black women (displayed in chapter 7, table 7–2). Hispanic and Asian women, however, are more likely to live with a spouse or with their children and grandchildren. This pattern is in contrast to whites and blacks who are from two to three times *less* likely to live with their children and grandchildren. Hispanic and Asian men are less likely to live alone than are the white and black men.

Number and Sex of Living Children. Given the economic, emotional, and social support that a spouse may have provided, children become particularly important for the partnerless elderly. An initial step to understanding these complex relationships beween parent and child is to first see how many children are available to the elder. Paul Glick (1977) found that in the United States, the eighty-year average of the average number of children was 3.18. Ethel Shanas (1977) found approximately four of every five persons sixty-five and older have at least one surviving child, while three-quarters have two or more.

We found among the white and black CSS respondents a higher incidence of childlessness than among the Hispanics and Asians (displayed in chapter 7, table 7–2). The childless rate is particularly high among blacks, both men and women, and among white men. If the childless were also spouseless then they may represent a particularly "at risk" group. On the average, however, the mean number of children for whites and blacks is slightly less than Glick's eighty-year average and slightly more among the Hispanics and Asians.

Given the traditional roles of women in American society, women are seen as principal caregivers. Consequently, the gender of the chidren is an important variable. Table 4–2 presents the mean number of children, by gender, of CSS respondents who have children. Although Hispanics and Asians have, on the average, more daughters than whites and blacks this appears to be a result of simply having more children.

In addition to gender, the child's marital status may affect his or her availability to lend assistance. Given the average age of our CSS respondents (seventy-five years old), this means that the "child" is in his or her fifties, a time of "emptying the nest." So, even if the daughter is married, some discretionary time may be available for the parent. As we saw from Gertrude's story, her daughter, Marge, spent a tremendous amount of time with her, both physically and on the telephone. Ethel Shanas (1977) found about 75 percent of the daughters are married. We found a slightly lower rate and significant variation among ethnic and racial groupings (table 4–3). For example, over 80 percent of the Asian daughters are married, while only slightly more than 50 percent of the black daughters are married.

Proximity of Children. As was true for Gertrude, most of the low-income elderly live near their children (table 4–4). If the number of CSS respondents who lived in the same house as their children were removed from table 4–4, the percentage would still be high.

Table 4–2
Mean number of sons and daughters, by ethnic/racial group and by gender

				Ethnic/Racial Groups[a]				
	White		*Black*		*Hispanic*		*Asian*[b]	
	Male	*Female*	*Male*	*Female*	*Male*	*Female*	*Male*	*Female*
Children	*(n=159)*	*(n=477)*	*(n=41)*	*(n=104)*	*(n=26)*	*(n=79)*	*(n=31)*	*(n=67)*
Sons	0.8	0.9	1.0	0.7	1.7	1.7	1.7	1.5
Daughters	0.8	1.0	0.9	0.9	1.8	1.5	1.5	1.4

[a]Other groupings, such as American Indian and Filipinos, were excluded because of small cell sizes.
[b]"Asian" includes Chinese, Japanese, and Korean.

Table 4–3
Percentage distribution of married sons and daughters, by ethnic/racial group and by gender

	White		Black		Hispanic		Asian[b]	
Presently Married	Male (n=159)	Female (n=477)	Male (n=41)	Female (n=104)	Male (n=26)	Female (n=79)	Male (n=31)	Female (n=67)
Sons: Yes	75	71	56	57	66	68	73	89
Daughters: Yes	63	64	56	54	57	67	82	81

[a]Other groupings, such as American Indian and Filipinos, were excluded because of small cell sizes.
[b]"Asian" includes Chinese, Japanese, and Korean.

The tendency to maintain separate households but live close by was first reported over forty years ago by Joseph Sheldon (1948) in England. Termed "intimacy at a distance" by Leopold Rosenmayr and Eva Köckeis (1963), the pattern still holds true for our low-income sample. As Rosenmayr and Köckeis point out, this preference exists in all European countries studied, as well as in the United States. Ethel Shanas (1977) reported that about half the elderly lived within a thirty-minute journey of their nearest child. Some theorists posit that the pattern evolved once the family ceased to be a unit of production.

In Gertrude's case, the desire for independence and autonomy was so strong that she kept secret from her duaghter her fall from bed. She simply did not want to move in with Marge, the loving, caring daughter. This attitude seems to hold true in all Western industrial countries, regardless of socioeconomic status or ethnic grouping.

Grandchildren, Great-grandchildren, and Siblings. To round out this description of low-income elderly's family structure, we present data on the number of grandchildren, great-grandchildren, and siblings. In table 4–1, "Number

Table 4–4
Percentage distribution of proximity of children, by ethnic/racial group and by gender

	White		Black		Hispanic		Asian[b]	
Proximity	Male (n=159)	Female (n=477)	Male (n=41)	Female (n=104)	Male (n=26)	Female (n=79)	Male (n=31)	Female (n=67)
Same house	7	10	15	21	9	23	11	33
Within 1 hour	46	50	56	49	55	44	39	42
More than 1 hour	47	40	29	30	36	33	50	25

[a]Other groupings, such as American Indian and Filipinos, were excluded because of small cell sizes.
[b]"Asian" includes Chinese, Japanese, and Korean.

of Generations", we see that over half the CSS respondents belong to three- and four-generation families. Data in chapter 7 (table 7–2) display the mean number of grandchildren for those CSS respondents with children. The relatively large numbers of grandchildren, ranging from a low of 6.0 for white men to a high of 14.2 for Hispanic women indicate the robustness of the family structure of those with children. All told, 86 percent of the respondents with children have grandchildren.

Summary. The family structure of the low-income elderly differs from the elderly in general in the state of spouselessness and living alone. The poor elderly seem similar to their more affluent peers in terms of number of children and grandchildren and that the children live nearby. We now turn to the nature of the interactions between parents and children.

Family Interactions

Frequency of Contact. Children frequently contact their parents (a "contact" can be face-to-face, a telephone call, or a letter). About 88 percent of the CSS respondents who report having children say that they have had a contact within the last week (table 4–5). Over half report a contact "today or yesterday." Marge, Gertrude's daughter, called twice a day and once at exactly 2:45 P.M. to check in.

Assistance Patterns. The CSS questionnaire contains a section dealing with nineteen areas of possible assistance the elder receives. These areas range from such personal care tasks as bathing and toileting to general care, or

Table 4–5
Percentage distribution of frequency of contact by children, by ethnic/racial group and by gender

	White		Black		Hispanic		Asian[b]	
Frequency	Male (n=143)	Female (n=451)	Male (n=41)	Female (n=98)	Male (n=26)	Female (n=77)	Male (n=31)	Female (n=67)
Today, yesterday	43	56	58	68	81	78	39	54
2–7 days ago	27	29	15	16	11	13	29	37
8–30 days ago	10	8	15	12	0	4	13	5
Over 30 days ago	20	7	12	3	8	5	19	5

[a]Other groupings, such as American Indian and Filipinos, were excluded because of small cell sizes.
[b]"Asian" includes Chinese, Japanese, and Korean.

instrumental tasks, such as laundry and home repair. The respondent was asked about each area and the research assistant coded the responses in one of five ways:

1. Respondent says does need assistance and gets support from family and/or friends;
2. Respondent says does not need assistance;
3. Respondent says does not have assistance but needs support;
4. Respondent says assistance provided by other than family and/or friends; and
5. Not applicable.

No combination responses were permitted and when faced with a combination response, the CSS research assistants were instructed to probe and code the *primary* source of assistance.

No Assistance Received or Needed.

Somewhat unexpectedly, we found a general pattern of self-sufficiency (table 4–6). Personal assistance is received by most of at least one gender and ethnic group in only six categories: travel, shopping, meal preparation, laundry, housework, and home repair. In contrast to help received in these tasks, which are relatively strenuous, require some degree of manual dexterity and mobility and are instrumental rather than personal, there is a high degree of self-sufficiency in personal care tasks such as dressing and bathing.

Assistance Received.

When we look at those who do receive assistance, from whatever source, we find that as age increases so does the number of areas in which assistance is received (table 4–7). Although this is expected, what may be surprising is the relative need in all age groups. All told, only 21 percent of the entire sample report receiving no assistance. The youngest male group, sixty-five to seventy-four, reports only 33 percent receiving no assistance and the youngest female group, sixty-five to seventy-four, reports only 24 percent receiving no assistance. For the oldest group, eighty-five and older, 15 percent of the men and only 6 percent of the women report no assistance. No substantitive difference appears to exist between the sexes.

The concept of "age as the great leveler" can be seen very clearly in this table. The average number of areas of assistance of all respondents rises from 3.0 for the sixty-five- to-seventy-four-years-old age group, to 4.2 for the seventy-five- to-eighty-four-years-old age group, and to 6.3 for the eighty-

Table 4–6

Percentage distribution of CSS participants reporting no assistance received or needed, by ethnic/racial group and gender

Area of Assistance	Ethnic/Racial Groups[a]							
	White		Black		Hispanic		Asian[b]	
	Male (n=235)	Female (n=614)	Male (n=71)	Female (n=168)	Male (n=32)	Female (n=97)	Male (n=37)	Female (n=69)
Personal care:								
Eating	92	90	93	92	100	96	95	96
Toileting	92	89	94	92	100	93	92	96
Transfer	92	88	94	92	97	93	95	91
Dressing	89	85	93	84	100	89	95	94
Walking	88	83	90	86	97	90	84	91
Bathing	79	79	82	76	91	85	81	84
Medicines	72	76	80	80	69	81	81	77
Instrumental care:								
Phoning	83	85	89	80	94	78	78	67
Out. Mob.	80	67	83	62	94	67	81	70
Stairs	77	74	76	65	88	83	89	80
Money Mgt.	75	71	73	70	75	72	73	54
Soc. Netwk.	75	64	69	62	78	53	81	68
Accomp.	68	58	76	57	78	50	84	59
Travel	67	**48**	73	**46**	78	54	73	**44**
Shopping	54	**41**	56	**38**	53	**41**	65	**39**
Meal Prep.	**49**	69	54	68	**38**	69	51	64
Laundry	**48**	52	**41**	**47**	**31**	55	**46**	**49**
Housewk.	**43**	**46**	**48**	**48**	**34**	54	**49**	55
Home Repair	**41**	**27**	**34**	**33**	**44**	**29**	78	55

[a]Other groupings, such as American Indian and Filipinos, were excluded because of small cell sizes.
[b]"Asian" includes Chinese, Japanese, and Korean.
[c]Those tasks for which a majority reported receiving assistance are in bold.

five-and-older group. The gender-specific patterns also show this increase in assistance as the respondents are older.

This pattern of assistance received is higher than the general elderly population as reported by Shanas (1977) and may reflect a lifelong correlation between lower socioeconomic status and increased morbidity rates.

Source of Assistance.

Of those who do receive personal assistance we found that family and friends (the "informal system") supply most of it and the system of publicly funded services (the "formal" system) supplies the smaller share (table 4–8). Because the CSS respondents are all SSI/SSP recipients and are receiving Medicaid, we do not believe this reliance on the informal support system is because of lack of access to public services. The CSS respondents are tied into "the system" but whether that "system" has sufficient level of services for the need is another question.

Table 4–7
Number of areas of assistance received, by age group and gender

Number of Areas	Male 65–74 (n=226)	75–85 (n=153)	85+ (n=46)	Female 65–74 (n=439)	75–84 (n=395)	85+ (n=178)
0	74	37	7	105	70	11
1	31	7	3	93	59	13
2	19	16	3	45	35	11
3	23	17	2	38	27	9
4	21	14	3	36	41	11
5	18	7	5	26	26	12
6	10	7	2	15	16	11
7	4	13	4	17	20	11
8	4	7	7	14	22	11
9	5	4	0	11	26	9
10+	17	24	10	39	53	69
Total Respondents	226	153	46	439	395	178
Mean (All)	2.9	4.2	5.4	3.2	4.2	6.5
Mean (Receivers only)	4.3	5.6	6.4	4.1	5.1	6.9

Table 4–8
Proportion of assistance received from the informal or formal support system, by gender

Assistance Area	Male Informal/Formal (%)	(%)	Female Informal/Formal (%)	(%)
Personal Care:				
Eating	55.0	45.0	41.8	58.2
Bathing	55.2	44.8	44.0	56.0
Transfer	47.1	52.9	40.0	60.0
Walking	59.3	40.7	53.9	46.1
Toileting	57.9	42.1	38.1	61.9
Dressing	60.7	39.3	46.9	53.1
Medications	50.9	49.1	44.9	55.1
Instrumental Care:				
Laundry	65.7	34.3	53.6	46.4
Phoning	72.5	27.5	65.9	34.1
Money Mgt.	85.3	14.7	84.7	15.3
Travel	75.3	24.7	77.8	22.2
Shopping	74.3	25.7	71.9	28.1
Housework	64.8	35.2	45.9	54.1
Meal Prep.	70.0	30.0	47.6	52.4
Outside Mobility	61.7	38.3	68.6	31.4
Stairclimbing	63.2	36.8	68.2	31.8
Social Network	87.0	13.0	83.0	17.0
Accompanying	71.3	28.7	71.7	28.3
Home Repair	21.6	78.4	34.2	65.8

On the other hand, CSS respondents do use both systems of support concurrently. This pattern directly contradicts Toni Antonucci's (1985) observation that research evidence suggests that, for the most part, the frail elderly receive either formal or informal supports, but not both. Gertrude Aston received assistance from the county-supplied In-Home Supportive Services worker while her daughter checked in by telephone, provided transport to the doctor, and helped with the grocery shopping. More generally, our data in table 4–8 indicate that both systems operate together in a functional manner for most of our low-income sample. The systems should be seen more as a dyad than as a mutually exclusive dichotomy.

Although overall, the CSS respondents rely on the informal support system for care, gender-specific differences exist. This can be seen most clearly in the areas of personal care. In these seven areas most women receive this assistance from the formal system, while most men receive this assistance from the informal system. Several things may explain this difference. First, as we shall see in the following section, the spouse is the primary provider of assistance within the informal support network. Because men have a shorter life expectancy than women, men are more likely to have a spouse taking care of them until they die. The reverse is true for women in that they will outlive their caring spouses. Second, anecdotal reports from social workers who actually arrange services for the elderly indicate that the man is less likely to acknowledge the existence of a personal care "need" than is the woman. Apparently, machismo proudly continues until the grave.

The greatest proportionate use of formal services by both sexes is for home repairs. When provided, this assistance is usually given by a landlord, not by a public service agency.

Results in table 4–8 point out severe limitations in the two current theoretical constructs that describe these overall patterns of caregiving and that attempt to explain from which system the elderly receive assistance. The two major models are the task-specific model (Cantor 1979) and the hierarchical compensatory model (Shanas 1979b). In the task-specific model, support is ordered by the nature of the task and the characteristics of the caregiver. Judith Sangl (1985) summarizes the theory as follows:

> According to this theory, kin are the most appropriate for tasks that require long-term involvement and intimacy.
>
> Neighbors would perform those tasks that require speed of response, knowledge and proximity to the living situation. Friends would be able to handle matters relating to peer group status and similarity of experience, such as sharing social activities.

Sangl goes on to summarize the hierarchical-compensatory model (Shanas, 1979b) as one in which:

Support is ordered according to the primacy of the relationship of the support given to the elderly recipient rather than to the nature of the task. In cases in which the initially preferred element is absent, other groups act in a compensatory manner as replacements.

Although we can see elements of both theories in operation, there is a major exception. Neither theory takes into consideration the economic status of the elderly and the availability of publicly funded services for low-income elderly. Cantor's original sample, upon which her constructs are built, was from a low-income population but gathered before the time when social services were widely available. For example, Title XX of the Social Security Act, a primary funding source for social services to the elderly, was not passed until 1975. Medicaid-funded home health aide services were also not widely available until recently.

Ironically, publicly funded services are not as available to middle-class elderly as they are to the low-income groups, such as our CSS Medicaid eligible sample. Middle-class elderly do not have sufficient disposable income to pay out-of-pocket expenses for these kinds of services. Barbara Silverstone (1985) points out that higher socioeconomic groups tend to have a greater use of formal services, which suggests that the use pattern of formal services by socioeconomic groups may be in the form of a U-shaped curve. The y-axis in this case would be the level of formal services and the x-axis would be socioeconomic groups.

Our CSS data show that when publicly funded services are available, they are used for precisely those kinds of services the task-specific model would predict to be supplied by kin: tasks that require long-term involvement and intimacy, the personal care tasks of table 4–8. Our data show that this type of assistance is provided through the county-supplied In-Home Supportive Services worker.

This reliance by our CSS women on the formal system for personal care tasks also is counter to what the hierarchical compensatory model would predict. This model posits that if the initially preferred element (the spouse) is missing, then other groups (such as daughters) compensate as replacements. In the CSS case, the "initially preferred element" would be the husband and then the daughter as a compensatory replacement. We know that most of the women are spouseless but that their daughters are very much present (tables 4–2, 4–3, 4–4, and 4–5). Also, we shall see later that in the areas of instrumental care, the daughters are the primary source of assistance. There is no indication the daughters are missing or unwilling to help, yet the formal system provides most of the help in the areas of personal care.

We shall examine the use of informal support in a multivariate framework later in this chapter, but suffice to say that sex, money, and formal service availability are variables that should not be underestimated when trying to understand the dynamics of the informal support system.

Informal Providers. We found that the spouse and then the daughter were the principal providers of informal care. For those CSS respondents who were married and received assistance, it was the spouse who provided the assistance. For the spouseless respondents, daughters provided most of the care.

Data in table 4–9 dramatically illustrate the synergistic relationship between spouses. In all but one case, "travel" for the married men it was the wife or husband who provided the assistance. We do not know who provided assistance to the married men. The answer to the question, "Will you still need me, will you still feed me, when I'm sixty-four?" is a resounding "Yes," if the two are still together.

For the spouseless, the patterns are different. The main source of assistance is the daughter. For spouseless women, the daughter is the primary source for almost all areas, with the friend as the primary source for travel. This was very much the case with Gertrude in that Marge, the daughter, would help with shopping, monthly checkups with the physician, and weekly meals. Gertrude's friend, Mrs. Smythe, travels with her when they frequent Pier 39 and people-watch.

For the spouseless man, the daughter also is the primary source for assistance, but the friend plays a major role, much more so than for the spouseless female. In the eight areas of instrumental care the friend is the primary source for five. This may reflect the pattern of greater incidence of childlessness among the men, particularly the black men, that we saw in table 4–4.

Overall, when examining the patterns of just the informal support system, there seems to be division of labor that first uses the spouse as primary source of assistance, then the daughter, then the friend. In this case, the informal support system alone fits the hierarchical compensatory model better than the task-specific model.

Reciprocity or Duty. After reviewing these assistance patterns, particularly the extensive help provided by the children, a question arises. Do they perform these tasks "as my duty bids," as Cordelia told her father, or as a component of reciprocity? Shanas (1977) states that it is the latter:

> Today family relations between the elderly and their children are more reciprocal in nature than they were 13 years ago [1963 to 1975]. These relations are less likely to be characterized by dutiful assistance on the part of adult children.

CSS data suggest this is *not* the case among the poor California elderly and their children. Duty or other motivational factors play a larger role than had been observed by Shanas. This statement is based on comparing similar

Table 4–9
Average number of providers of informal care for CSS respondents receiving informal care, by gender and marital status (most frequently mentioned provider in parentheses)

	Male		Female	
Task	Married (n=138)	Spouseless (n=178)	Married (n=104)	Spouseless (n–698)
Personal care:				
Eating	1.0 (Spouse)	1.0 (Daughter)	1.3 (Spouse)	1.1 (Daughter)
Toileting	1.0 (Spouse)	1.0 (Daughter)	1.5 (Spouse)	1.2 (Daughter)
Transfer[a]	1.2 (Spouse)	n/a n/a	1.3 (Spouse)	3.3 (Daughter)
Dressing	1.1 (Spouse)	1.2 (Daughter)	1.3 (Spouse)	1.0 (Daughter)
Walking	1.7 (Spouse)	1.9 (Friend)	1.5 (Spouse)	1.4 (Daughter)
Bathing	1.0 (Spouse)	1.0 (Daughter)	1.2 (Spouse)	1.2 (Daughter)
Foot Care	2.1 (Spouse)	1.0 (Daughter)	1.0 (Daughter)	1,0 (Daughter)
Grooming	1.0 (Spouse)	1.0 (Daughter)	1.0 (Spouse)	1.0 (Daughter)
Instrumental care:				
Phoning	1.1 (Spouse)	1.0 (Daughter)	1.1 (Spouse)	1.2 (Daughter)
Stairs	1.0 (Spouse)	1.3 (Friend)	1.4 (Spouse)	1.5 (Daughter)
Money Mgt.	1.0 (Spouse)	1.0 (Daughter)	1.1 (Spouse)	1.1 (Daughter)
Travel	1.1 (Daughter/Son)	1.3 (Friend)	1.4 (Spouse)	1.5 (Friend)
Shopping	1.4 (Spouse)	1.0 (Friend)	1.1 (Spouse)	1.1 (Daughter)
Meal Prep.	1.2 (Spouse)	1.0 (Friend)	1.1 (Spouse)	1.1 (Daughter)
Laundry	1.2 (Spouse)	1.0 (Friend)	1.1 (Spouse)	1.0 (Daughter)
Housework	1.3 (Spouse)	1.0 (Daughter)	1.2 (Spouse)	1.1 (Daughter)

[a]In the case of transfer for spouseless males the "n/a" means there were no spouseless males receiving assistance in transfer.

items between the two surveys that ask about what kinds of assistance respondents provide their children. The results in table 4–9 are presented in terms of percentages of those who said, yes, they do provide the specific kind of assistance. Data are from the National Survey by Shanas (1977, table 7–19A).

The magnitude of differences, two and three times as great and all statistically significant, between the two surveys strongly suggests that among the poor California elderly, children's care for their parent(s) is not dominantly characterized by reciprocity, at least not an immediate tit-for-tat type of reciprocity.

The reciprocity patterns shown in table 4–10 also cast some doubts about the appropriateness of a social exchange theory to explain filial responsibilities. Marvin Sussman (1985) goes so far as to posit that those who carry out these responsibilities expect to receive more than their legal share of any inheritance, a type of "those who do, will receive." Keeping in mind that our CSS respondents are all poor, with a legal maximum as to the amount of real and personal property that they may possess, an expectation of inheritance cannot be a strong motivational factor for their helpful children. In addition, under California law, if a Medicaid recipient should happen to leave an "estate," the Medicaid program has first claim to it.

One of the familial dimensions that Gertrude's story highlights, not captured by our survey data, is the dynamic nature of family relationships and how they change over time. For example, when Gertrude's grandchildren were infants, Gertrude was actively and intensely involved in their care to the point that they would crawl out of bed and sleep outside her door just to be closer to her. Now, at age ninety, the direction of assistance is reversed.

Table 4–10
Reciprocity patterns among "National Survey" respondents and CSS respondents toward their children

Specific Kind of Assistance Provided	National Survey			CSS		
	Men (n=832) %	Women (n=1,256) %	All (n=2,089) %	Men (n=292) %	Women (n=760) %	All (n=1,052) %
Gifts to children or to their families	75	65	69	46	50	49
Caring for grandchildren	28	41	36	18	18	18
Home repair for children	24	3	11	8	2	4
Housekeeping for children	11	39	28	5	11	10

In this context, reciprocity is more a lifetime concept, and the givers and receivers change roles over the years, although never completely abandoning the duality of roles. Only the proportionate shares change.

Multivariate Analyses

Explaining and Predicting Contact by Children. To better understand the dynamics of contact by children with their parents we carried out a series of regression analyses. We ultimately constructed a model containing 28 independent variables and explaining 21 percent of the variance (results are shown in table 4–11). The statistically significant variables that explain and predict the frequency of contact by children are as follows:

More Contact	*Less Contact*
• Number of children	• Male
• More informal support	• Living alone
	• More siblings
	• More grandchildren

What this means is that as one has more children, one has more contact. This term, when squared, was also statistically significant and negative, which means that as the number of children increases, the additional contact

Table 4–11
**Regression results with frequency of contact by children
as the dependent variable**

Variable	Parameter Estimate	Probability That Parameter = 0
Intercept	2.733962	0.0006
Sex (1 = male; 0 = female)	−0.513276	0.0001
Living alone	−0.295595	0.0004
Number of siblings^2	−0.00874738	0.0616
Number of children	0.240913	0.0001
Number of children^2	−0.0130012	0.0077
Number of grandchildren	−0.021791	0.0393
Number of informal help areas	0.133145	0.0001
Number of informal help areas^2	−0.00610713	0.0161

$^p \leq 0.10$; $r^2 = 0.2476$; adjusted $r^2 = 0.2097$

Other variables tested but not significant at the 0.10 level were age, race, educational level, hearing status, vision status, number of dangerous diseases (i.e., cancer, diabetes, stroke, asthma, hardening of arteries, heart trouble, high blood pressure, and kidney/bladder disease), ADL level, ADL level squared, IADL level, IADL level squared, mental status impairment level, mental status impairment level squared, number of formal services received, number of formal services received squared, the number of siblings, the number of grandchildren squared, and self-reported health status of "poor."

increases at a slower rate. And, the more informal support, the more contact. As we saw in table 4–9, the daughter is a primary source of informal support, so we would expect this relationship. Less contact by children is associated with being a man and living alone. The man seems to be more estranged from his children than does the woman, which may be attributable to a lifelong distancing process. That living alone is negatively associated with contact is a puzzlement that has no immediate intuitive explanation. A speculation is that those who live alone may prefer this situation and avoid contact.

That more siblings and more grandchildren are negatively associated with contact could be an expression of a division of labor and/or that the child with many children does not have as much extra time for parent contact.

The variables that did not prove to be statistically significant were also interesting. No statistically significant differences were associated with racial or ethnic grouping, with measures of functional or mental impairment, with the number of formal services received, or with age. Contact by children seems to occur universally without regard to some perception of increased "need," and it did not decrease in the presence of formal services. This was certainly the case for Gertrude with her daughter's daily contact, even though the county-supplied chore worker came to her apartment five days a week.

Explaining and Predicting Informal Support. Who is more likely to receive informal support from among our CSS and what are the determinants of receiving more help? These are the questions we analyzed through multivariate regression, the results of which are shown in table 4–12. Using a model constructed with twenty-eight independent variables, we were able to explain 67 percent of the variance, a particularly high level of explanation in the field of social science research. This finding confirms an earlier and similar analysis carried out independently but achieving almost exactly the same level of explanation (Pelham and Clark 1983). The statistically significant variables of the present analysis explaining and predicting the receipt of informal support are as follows:

More Informal Help	*Less Informal Help*
• Number of siblings	• Female
• Number of children	• "Other" racial (e.g., Asian)
• "Poor" health status	• Higher ADL score
• Contact	• Higher IADL score
	• Formal services

Overall, those who get informal help are those who need personal assistance in carrying out everyday tasks (i.e., low Activities of Daily Living score and low Instrumental Activities of Living score), and are sickly (i.e., a self-

Table 4–12
Regression results with the number of areas of support provided
by the informal support system as the dependent variable

Variable	Parameter Estimate	Probability That Parameter = 0
Intercept	13.324238	0.0001
Sex (1 = male; 0 = female)	−0.487187	0.0034
"Other" racial (e.g., Asian)	−0.340145	0.0960
ADL Independencies	−1.038452	0.0315
IADL Independencies	−0.702233	0.0001
IADL Independencies^2	−0.056139	0.0012
Number of formal services	−0.855031	0.0001
Number of formal services^2	0.012128	0.0149
Number of siblings	0.260693	0.0002
Number of siblings^2	−0.038898	0.0001
Number of children	0.135182	0.0818
Poor health status	0.331001	0.0742
Frequency of children contact	0.570566	0.0110
Frequency of children contact^2	−0.115041	0.0191

$p \leq 0.10$
$r^2 = 0.6768$; adjusted $r^2 = 0.6682$
Other variables tested but not significant at the 0.10 level were age, living alone, race, educational level, hearing status, vision status, number of dangerous diseases (i.e., cancer, diabetes, stroke, asthma, hardening of arteries, heart trouble, high blood pressure, and kidney/bladder disease), ADL level squared, IADL level squared, mental status impairment level, mental status impairment level squared, the number of siblings squared, the number of grandchildren, and the number of grandchildren squared.

reported health status of "poor"), are males, and have family members to provide the support if formal services are not being used. That men receive more assistance than women may be the result of a cultural and gender-specific "learned helplessness" on the part of the man and the ascribed role of the woman as the care provider. Also, it may be that women are relatively stronger than men at this advanced age.

From a policy point of view, an important finding is that as the number of formal services goes up, the number of informal areas goes down, although, as the squared term of formal services indicates, this relationship decreases or levels off as the number of formal services are higher. This substitution of informal by formal is what we first saw in table 4–8, "Proportion of assistance received from the informal or formal support system, by gender." What we saw there was increased use of formal services for the personal care tasks on the part of women. What the present analysis shows is that each additional formal service is associated with a decrease of 0.8 informally supported tasks. Most likely, given the results of table 4–8, those services to be substituted are the personal care kind, also referred to as the "Activities of Daily Living."

Of those variables that were not statistically significant, perhaps the most interesting was *age,* indicating that age per se may not be the best criterion for assessing individual need. The effect we saw in table 4–7, "Number of areas of assistance received, by age group and gender," in which the average number of areas of assistance received increased by age group, may be more properly seen as a cohort effect rather than as a person-specific effect. Age, in the long run, is certainly a "leveler," but it happens at a very uneven rate at the individual level.

Adaptations to the Need for Help

What emerges from these data showing personal and instrumental self-sufficiency and the relatively high incidence of debilitating chronic conditions, discussed in chapters 5 and 6, is a pattern of adaptation (Pelham 1980). For example, table 4–6 shows little assistance reported for stair climbing because respondents say they avoid climbing stairs.

A similar example is outside mobility in that respondents state that they do not go out as often as they used to. In addition, some respondents reported that, although they do not require personal assistance in bathing, they will not bathe unless someone else is present in the house for fear of falling while alone. Conversely, laundry and shopping are areas of relatively high levels of assistance, but are of such a nature that they cannot be deleted from the daily tasks of life. Apparently, the poor elderly choose to avoid tasks or adapt alternative means of performing them as a first preference, and then rely on others for assistance when there is not an alternative. In other words, the poor elderly prefer autonomy at a cost of not participating in life as fully as they may have at an earlier age.

Policy Considerations

Policy makers have long recognized the value of the informal support system in providing care for the elderly and are concerned about the effects of public programs on that support system. Specifically, a primary concern is that as publicly funded services become more available, family care providers may abdicate their traditional familial responsibilities, resulting in an increase in the level of public expenditures. For example, among our CSS respondents, the most frequently used nonmedical service was In-Home Supportive Services (14 percent of the sample). That service, funded through the Social Services Block Grant of Title XX of the Social Security Act, provides a variety of personal care and housekeeping tasks to a functionally disabled population, including light or heavy housekeeping, shopping, and bathing. IHSS is now the largest single social service program in California and was funded during fiscal year 1983–84 at $0.3 billion with 96,850 recipients (California 1984). This represents an annual average cost per recipient of approximately

$3,070. The recipient population sixty-five and older (66,023) represents approximately just 3 percent of the total California elderly population and 19 percent of the low-income (SSI/SSP) population.

The single largest publicly funded social service program is reaching only about 19 percent of the poor elderly California population at a cost of almost one-third of a billion dollars. The informal support system is providing a similar kind of care to over half of the poor elderly population at no public cost. One begins to realize how valuable is the informal support system (chapter 6 describes and analyzes IHSS more fully).

What we have seen in our CSS data is that there does appear to be a substitution of informal by formal support in certain areas and that it is fairly predictable (i.e., about 1.0 formal for 0.8 informal). We have also seen that the areas of support most likely to be substituted are the personal care kind. Our personal observation is that when this phenomenon is discussed among advocates for aging programs, this substitution effect is minimized, dismissed, or mitigated by the claim for "more research," preferably more longitudinal studies. Given the fierce competition over scarce fiscal resources, this attitude is understandable but misleading in the long run. We suggest that the substitution effect be recognized for what it is: relief for the family care provider of *some* tasks. We have seen that the family, particularly women family members, is still very active in caring for the elderly despite the availability of publicly funded services. Program advocates may be more productive if their efforts were directed at changing the U-shaped curve so that formal services are more equitably accessible to the middle socioeconomic groups.

5
Functional Status

Agnes Hughes

Agnes Hughes is seventy-eight years old and has lived thirty years in a tall, old, wood frame house. It has one bedroom, kitchen, bath, "junk room," and living room. She says "Indians" originally built the house.

To get to Agnes' house, a visitor must first pass through a locked iron gate that is supposed to be unlocked by a set of buzzers inside the house. The buzzers do not work. The iron gate separates the street from an alley pathway to her house set in the back, behind the house facing the street. Like most San Francisco houses, the ones on Agnes' street are built flush; the exterior side walls of the houses are common. The gate door that does not operate locks Agnes in or out as the case may be. She must anticipate the arrival of guests and slowly descend stairs, cross a trash-heaped courtyard, feel her way through the dim alley, unlock the gate, and then wait.

Past the ratty stone courtyard is a steep flight of outdoor, creaking wooden stairs that have been painted and repainted. Indoors is a second, narrow flight of stairs that curves into an entry hall and kitchen. The walls are a combination of wood and plaster painted a greenish hue.

Agnes wears a hospital gown with a long sweater wrap, a nylon stocking hair cover, and gold-colored earrings. She is not in good health. Eight months ago she had bowel surgery. She suffers from a "burning" stomach (not pain, she explains), loss of appetite, and gas. She has a hernia in the chest area. Last year she had a hip replacement. To date she has had three hip replacements, two on the right side and one of the left. She underwent surgery in 1983, 1984, and 1985.

She does not sleep well at night and she gets up "late" these days—8 A.M. She has no alarm clock and does not need one. When she wakes she fixes up her face and teeth, takes her medicines, and eats her All Bran for breakfast. She cooks her own meals and never has "idle hands." Her eating and feeding abilities are functionally adequate. Also, she manages her toileting and dressing adequately.

This week she began taking acupuncture for pain. Taxi vouchers take her to a Chinese College Medical Center. The acupuncture seems to have diminished her pain already. Her case manager, Brenda, from a local, community-based, long-term care agency, made arrangements for the alternative medical intervention to control the pain. Agnes says acupuncture needles cause no great pain themselves, "except for like a shot." She has to use her Medi-Cal "Proof of Eligibility" stickers (coin of the realm for medical services through the Medicaid program) but only gets five stickers a month. She doesn't seem to know that she can get more if she needs them.

She uses a cane outdoors. While inside the house, she turns on the burners of the gas stove for extra heat. She has a huge old wooden bed, linoleum floors, and a little radio tuned to religious programs.

Agnes' philosophy of life is belief in self-reliance. "Yes, sir. Use your own head—not the views of others. Look to God and you'll come out all right." As a black woman, Agnes says she never suffered any racial discrimination. "If you don't use your own head, who's going to use it?" She was always very polite, however. "Don't think that you are white because you're not. You have to use your head and put God first in your life."

She is a member of the Pentecostal Church and has been for thirty years, but she does not go to church as much now. The church is just around the corner. She explains she is a Christian and that means "Christlike." She further explains she is not "religious" but Christian. She says, "'Christian' means that you are saved and filled with the Holy Spirit. That's the difference between being Christian and being religious."

Agnes was born in Mississippi and raised in Baton Rouge, Louisiana. She met her husband in Mississippi and later divorced. He has since died. Agnes, born on a farm, worked in the fields, picked cotton, dug potatoes, picked peanuts, and pulled corn.

She attended school all day, then went to the fields. She made it to the ninth grade and knows that she is better educated than the twelfth-graders of today.

Her family owned a farm on the Nichols plantation. Her chore was to milk the cow in the morning and in the evening. The Nichols family lived in the big house. They were white. She remembers them well and they were good. Children of both families picked pecans together. The Nichols' dog's name was Loud. She was afraid of the dog because he barked like crazy. Agnes said, "His 'whop whop' bark could make you climb a tree backwards, let you know you're on the boss man's property." One sad memory of her childhood was the day her baby brother died.

She recalls that her family managed during the Depression. They grew their own food—hogs, goats, chickens, guinea hens. Agnes explains that guinea hens are speckled birds and, like dogs, they know when a stranger is approaching. They have long-shaped eggs, different from chickens. Agnes misses them.

During World War II Agnes found herself raising a son alone in Baton Rouge, Louisiana. She earned so little money she could not buy anything, so she sent him home to her parents in Mississippi for food and care. She continued to work alone in Baton Rouge and received $2.50 a week in the late 1930s.

Today Agnes has no family. Her one child died eleven years ago at age fifty-two of heart disease. Her son's name was Matt—"He never made my heart ache." He came to San Francisco after serving in the Army and he went back to the South to bring Agnes to San Francisco to live with him. She did not want to go because there were no porches or porch swings, and she did not have any friends in the West. She did not live with him, but he moved her into the house in which she has resided ever since.

Agnes' son had two sons, who she helped to raise. She cared for the boys until they were eleven and thirteen. Her son was divorced and when he remarried the grandchildren stayed with Agnes for a while. They then moved back to live with their own mother in Louisiana. Agnes had a woman in the neighborhood care for the boys during the day while she worked as a domestic and then would pick them up in the evening. The grandsons are now in their late twenties and early thirties.

Once a year at Christmas time the boys' mother will call. Their stepmother, the son's second wife, calls about once a month around the first and Agnes calls her toward the end of the month. Agnes has one adult brother still living in Mississippi. She recalls that she had four uncles and four aunts back in the old days on the farm.

Agnes worked until 1974 as a domestic. People she worked for are still "true friends," she says. They keep in touch and send checks on her birthday and at Christmas. She worked for two or three families between 1954 and 1974 as a domestic. She also worked back in Louisiana as a domestic and everybody she has worked for was "good" to her.

Today, she manages her own money. She mails her own telephone bill and carries the utility bill to a friend who then pays it for her. Remedy, Inc., a home health and In-Home Supportive Services agency supplied by the county, pays an escort to cash her check.

Twice a week a chore worker comes from Remedy, Inc., to clean, purchase groceries, and bathe Agnes. She works from 9:00 A.M. to 3:30 P.M., and takes the bus to the store because there are no supermarkets in the area. Agnes is simply not strong enough to make a trip on the bus to the market and return home with the grocery bags using her cane.

Agnes does her own dishes and light housekeeping but cannot get into or out of the tub alone. However, she can bathe the front of herself; the worker washes her back, feet, and hair. Agnes likes her chore worker and believes she is a caring, faithful helper.

Agnes still walks everywhere but does not travel by bus. She walks to Mt. Zion Hospital outpatient clinic once a month for a checkup and her medicine. She has a private doctor and she likes him. She would like to have a "lady doctor" but none are available.

Although Agnes is relatively alone, her daily living needs are met. With scant informal support system about, IHSS fills the gaps to meet her personal and housekeeping needs while the case manager coordinates the more bureaucratic processes. Agnes manages the remainder herself, such as it is. Contact with the outside world is mostly electronic: telephone, radio, television, and an occasional letter. The chore worker provides the primary human contact. Agnes has always kept a low profile so as not to create situations in which racial discrimination could occur. To this day she truly believes she suffered none.

However, Agnes says she feels discrimination today because she is old. She believes her faithful life's labor deserves a better old age. Money is the chief problem. She feels the government does not seem to care about the elderly.

Agnes is alone and cold a lot of the time. She dresses in ragged clothes. She cannot find an apartment on the flat and no one seems to be able to help. Agnes is not complaining—just making observations.

Introduction

The daily life of Agnes Hughes demonstrates the determination of most aged people to maintain their functional independence. Despite three surgeries in as many years, she independently performs her personal care activities, except for some assistance in bathing. In the more impersonal, sometimes called instrumental, activities, she needs help, partly because of her physical limitations and partly because of environmental circumstances.

For example, because of her hip surgery, she uses a cane. While that has not inhibited her mobility in many ways—she walks inside and out without assistance—she cannot shop because it requires a bus trip and perhaps carrying heavy groceries. But there is an environmental factor that also affects her functioning—the lack of stores nearby. If a market were available in the neighborhood, she might well not require assistance with most shopping. She needs help with the heavier housekeeping chores, but manages her meals, communications, and money without help.

After financial dependence, the problem most threatening to many of the aging population is the possible loss of functional ability. An acute medical problem, increasing weakness, or multiple chronic conditions can make the activities associated with independent living more and more difficult to perform. In addition to the practical problems of house cleaning, meals preparation, or bathing, there is the emotional problem of accepting diminished capabilities and increasing dependence on others.

Increased dependence is sometimes viewed as a return to the infantile state. The term "second childhood," often used jokingly to refer to age-inappropriate behavior, is a real fear to many aged persons. Being helped to eat or bathe or go to the toilet is a dreaded future for many. "Dying with one's boots on" implies not only avoiding the pain and worry of long illness, but avoiding the infantlike state of dependence often resulting from serious illness.

In this chapter we focus on the distribution of functional independence and dependence in the sample participating in the California Senior Survey.

Many of the public programs that provide services to the poor elderly deal directly with the results of functional dependence. For example, California's In-Home Supportive Services program serves SSI/SSP recipients who need help with the personal and instrumental activities of living. Title III funds provide meals, both in and out of home, to assure improved nutrition for people unable to prepare meals.

The community-based, long-term care programs sponsored by HCFA and based on a waiver from Medicaid now exist in almost all states. Medicaid funds in these programs can be used to pay for services in the home, most of which are necessary because of the recipients' need for help with daily living tasks.

These are only a few examples of myriad public and private programs whose primary purpose is to alleviate the problems of functional incapacity. (See chapter 6 for a more detailed description of services.) For all of them, one major concern is how to measure functional independence or dependence. Large-scale programs generally require some formal mechanism for demonstrating each client's need for their services.

Measuring Functional Status

There are a number of ways to describe functional status, depending upon the area of interest of the measurer. For example, physicians, nurses, or physical therapists may wish to evaluate functioning through precise measurements of the range of motion of arms, legs, and hands to prescribe particular therapies to help alleviate the functional loss. They also may want to measure functional change to assess the rate of recovery. These assessments may be particular to one body system or a more general measurement of functional capacity.

Some government agencies, most notably the Veterans Administration and the Social Security Administration, have based payments for disability on a schedule of diseases. Here, disability is measured by the particular condition, implying that certain degrees of functional dependence are the result of certain types of diseases or impairments. In general, this method can be a useful guide, but individual response to disease can cause marked differences in what different people afflicted with the same condition can or cannot do in their daily activities.

Social services agencies providing in-home care may be more interested in the implications of functional loss for performance of daily activities. That is, the measurement of range of motion in the arms is less helpful than the assessment of the person's ability to cook, clean, dress, and so forth. It is more efficient for assessment in these programs to measure the actual ability of a person to perform a particular task rather than try to apply the effects of range-of-motion limitations to tasks of daily living.

Researchers, assessors, and others have developed many scales or indexes to provide summary scores of functional ability in different dimensions. One dimension is mobility: the ability of an individual to move from one place to another, to be independent in transporting himself through his home and community. Another dimension consists of a set of personal care activities: bathing, dressing, toileting, continence, transfer, and eating. All these tasks are necessary to truly independent living.

A third set of daily activities consists of tasks that are generally termed instrumental. They are of a less personal but no less important nature. Among these activities, one of the more important and more frequently performed tasks is meal preparation. But other things must be done in the course of a safe and healthy independent existence: housecleaning, laundry, shopping, telephoning, transportation, money and medications management.

Another area is mental functioning. However physically well an individual, organic brain disease or mental illness can stand in the way of independence. Being able physically to cook a meal is only relevant if the person can remember to cook the meal, or can remember to turn off the burners afterward. The ability to judge the need for doing an activity or to judge the results of activities is part of independent functioning.

There are many measures of functioning in all these areas (Nagi 1969; Warski and Green 1971; Wright 1974; Wylie and White 1964). One constant problem in research of the disabled elderly is the multiplicity of measures, making comparisons between groups often difficult, ambiguous, or impossible. The California Senior Survey uses measures that are frequently used in both surveys and research studies. The Activities of Daily Living measure was developed by Dr. Sidney Katz and others (1963, 1970). It measures levels of independence in personal care activities. The Instrumental Activities of Daily Living is a comparable measure of independence is the less personal daily activities of living (Lawton and Brody 1969). The Short Portable Mental Status Questionnaire is an index of questions that test the time and place orientation of the respondent (Pfeiffer 1975). It measures the possible presence of organic brain disease.

All these measures have both a biological and environmental component. The biological component is the disease or condition that impairs the performance of an activity. The nature of the condition implies its effects upon daily living. A serious, but time-limited condition, such as a surgery for gall bladder removal indicates a major, but temporary, loss of functioning. The expectation would be that, barring complications, the individual could soon return to independent living. However, a stroke resulting in paralysis may mean that the individual will, for a long time if not permanently, require personal assistance in most daily activities.

The environmental component is the living area of the individual. It may be modified to provide aids to independence. Prosthetic devices and mechanical adjuncts, such as wheelchairs or safety bars in shower stalls, are examples of environmental modification. For many, such devices can delay or make personal help unnecessary. The environmental component is an area in which the poor are quite likely to suffer. There may not be resources to pay for modifying the living area. In many cases, where the individual rents living space, some modifications such as ramps or safety bars may not be available.

Activities of Daily Living

Walking

The ability to walk independently has ramifications for many other daily activities. Most tasks of daily living require a certain degree of mobility. If people are unable to walk independently, they may be able to do parts of daily chores, but be unable to complete the task. For example, a person may be able to sit at the table and peel vegetables or cut up meat for stew, but be unable to walk between sink and stove with a heavy pot. Bed-bound people may be able to feed themselves, but be unable to prepare the meal. A secondary result of lack of mobility is a lack of exercise, which tends to exacerbate any weakness. Table 5–1 shows the distribution of walking ability by the CSS participants.

In 1977, 1 percent of the noninstitutionalized aged population was reportedly bedridden (U.S. Department of Health, Education, and Welfare 1977). The data in table 5–1 show that a slightly higher percentage of California Senior Survey participants were bedridden than in the national sample. One and three-quarters percent of the females and less than 1 percent (0.64 percent) of the males were unable to move from their beds. However, as we

Table 5–1
Percentage distribution of mobility, by gender

Degree of mobility	Male		Female	
	Inside %	Outside %	Inside %	Outside %
Bedbound	0.60	0.63	1.72	1.72
Another person carries the individual	0.32	0.32	0.73	1.57
Walks with a mechanical device and help from another person	0.63	3.16	2.80	7.41
Walks with help from another person, but does not use mechanical devices	0.32	1.58	0.63	5.50
Walks with help from a mechanical device, but not from another person	18.20	25.00	17.22	22.90
Walks independent of mechanical supports or another person	79.90	69.31	76.90	60.90

see in the table, a substantial number of people did suffer some problem with mobility, although few needed personal help with ambulating. Approximately 23 percent of these women, like Alice Hughes, walk outdoors with help from mechanical devices, but without the help of another person.

Considering only inside mobility, 98 percent of the males and 94 percent of the females were able to ambulate without personal help. As people moved outdoors, both sexes required somewhat more help, both mechanical and personal.

Personal Care Activities

What have come to be known as the Activities of Daily Living are those tasks sometimes alternatively called personal care activities. The six tasks evaluated are bathing, eating, dressing, transfer, toileting, and continence. Although serious illness may abruptly cause temporary dependence in all six areas, recuperation often proceeds upon the same continuum as independence develops in a child (Katz et al. 1963). Recovery of independence in eating and continence usually come first. The patient then attains independence in transfer and toileting, dressing and bathing. Less precipitous loss of function because of increasing severity of chronic disease, in general, follows the reverse order. The first indication of decreasing independence is often the fear of or inability to bathe without personal help, followed by difficulties in dressing, transfer and toileting, continence and eating. These are, of course, general sequences of events; a particular illness may make the sequence different.

Figure 5–1 shows the distribution of independent functioning in the six

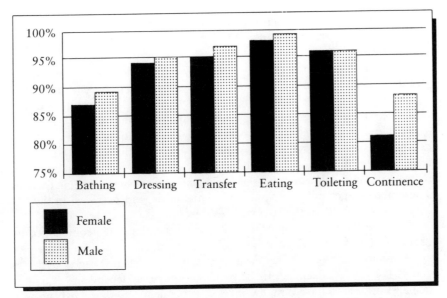

Figure 5-1. **Percentage of respondents independent in each activity of daily living**

Activities of Daily Living among the California Senior Survey participants, by sex. (Differences by age group are discussed in chapter 10.)

For both groups, the percentage of those who are independent in personal care activities is high. Independent in this study means independent of assistance from another person. If a person uses some device, but does not need personal help, he or she is considered independent. There is only a slight difference between men and women, with the men in this group exhibiting a somewhat higher level of independence in five of the six activities.

The most dependence for both groups occurs in continence care; the least in eating. About 19 percent of the women and 14 percent of the men need personal help with continence care. Only 2 percent of the women and 1 percent of the men report being unable to eat without personal assistance. While the differences for the most part are not significantly different, it is interesting to note that the males are consistently somewhat higher. A possible influence on the scores is suggested by discussions with case workers who interview the aged for in-home services. They note that men will sometimes report independence in personal care activities because they want to avoid help with these activities, particularly if the care provider is a woman.

Bathing is the task for which dependence is next most prevalent. As Agnes Hughes found, getting into and out of the tub can be hazardous; having another person nearby who can help is necessary. In chapter 10, we see that, predictably and especially for women, dependence increases in all areas as age increases. However, men who survive to join the ranks of the old-old (over eighty-five) also maintain their physical functioning to a greater degree than women.

Table 5–2 shows the dependencies between people in a national survey and the CSS participants. This comparison is based on only four of the ADL activities: bathing, dressing, eating, and toileting. It also separates the elderly into three often-used groupings, "young," "middle," and "old."

Table 5–2 data report a reasonable finding mentioned earlier: dependence increases as age increases. As population projections imply a relatively large increase in the population over eighty-five years old we can expect an increase in the absolute numbers of dependent persons in the coming decades. These percentages indicate a somewhat higher dependency level in the CSS Medicaid recipients in the two youngest groups.

Because this set of four ADL tasks includes eating, the people reporting dependence in four ADL tasks are quite disabled. As we saw in figure 5–1, approximately 2 percent of the entire CSS sample suffers this degree of dependency. For the less disabled, those reporting only one dependency, CSS participants appear to have a higher level of dependence, with the exception of the oldest group.

When all six items of the Activities of Daily Living are included, 81 percent of the females and 85 percent of the males were completely independent. Only 4 percent of the entire sample were dependent in three or more activities and there was no gender difference.

We have presented the results of the survey primarily in terms of the independence of the elderly in this sample. The obverse, dependency, and how it is measured may become more important in the future as a basis for payment of nursing home fees. Current experiments are using mobility and the ADL items, particularly dressing, as the indicator of service time required (Fries and Cooney 1985) for nursing home patients. For the minority of the poor elderly who are at risk of entering, or do enter, a nursing home, the measurement of functional dependence and of changes in that functioning will

Table 5–2
Percentage of persons reported as having some dependency in four Activities of Daily Living tasks, by age group

	Aged 65–74		Age 75–84		Age 85+	
Sample:	Nat'l %	CSS %	Nat'l %	CSS %	Nat'l %	CSS %
Dependent in:						
One ADL task	2.2	6.1	5.8	7.9	15.0	11.9
Four ADL tasks	0.4	0.5	0.6	1.3	3.7	3.6

National figures from Estes, Carroll L., *et al.*, *Political Economy, Health, and Aging* (Little Brown Series on Gerontology 1984).

determine the payment the nursing home receives. This may have as-yet-unknown affects upon nursing home entry and discharge.

A Multivariate Analysis of Personal Care Independence

The CSS participants were assessed on demographic, personal, and health variables. Table 5–3 shows the characteristics that were significantly associated with the degree of independence. The dependent variable in the regression anaysis was the sum of ADL items on which the individual was independent. The score can range from zero, meaning the person is completely dependent, to six, indicating independence on all personal care functions. The dependent variables were age, gender, amount of informal help, the sum

Table 5–3
Results of a regression of various personal characteristics on the sum of independent Activities of Daily Living

Variable	Unstandardized Parameter Estimate	Probability That Estimate Equals 0	Standardized Estimate
(Intercept)	5.5009	0.0001	
Aged 85+	0.0474	0.3098	0.0267
Male	0.0150	0.7714	0.0076
Amount of informal help	0.0172	0.0811	0.0638
Sum of IADL items	0.0572	0.0035	0.1273
Sum of correct SPMSQ	0.0324	0.0291	0.0594
Walks independently	0.1027	0.0624	0.0526
Rates health poor	−0.2251	0.0006	−0.0910
Life Satisfaction	0.0037	0.4441	0.0191
Black	−0.0272	0.6701	0.0111
Hispanic	−0.0439	0.5520	−0.0151
Other race (nonwhite)	0.0445	0.5040	0.0180
Lives alone	0.0055	0.9236	−0.0031
Married	−0.1138	0.0754	−0.0556
Educational level	−0.0321	0.2240	−0.0316
In bed in past two weeks	−0.0521	0.3757	−0.0221
Cut activities	0.1545	0.0073	0.0662
Hearing difficulties	0.0650	0.3247	0.0257
Vision difficulties	0.0449	0.4545	−0.0202
Number of serious chronic diseases	−0.2155	0.0001	−0.0964
Number of less serious chronic diseases	−0.0146	0.4462	−0.0231
Proportion of acute care in past six months	0.7001	0.3013	0.0253
Proportion of nursing home care in past six months	1.6598	0.0052	0.0686
Amount of help needed	−0.1074	0.0001	−0.5001

Adjusted R^2 = 0.4266, n = 1328
Variables whose parameter estimates are significant at p. ≤ 0.10 are in bold.

of the Instrumental Activities of Daily Living (discussed later), mobility, self-rated health, a measure of life satisfaction, race, living situation, marital status, education, past curtailment of activities, hearing and vision, chronic conditions or diseases, the proportion of time during the last six months that was spent in an acute care or nursing home institution.

The analysis is performed on the first assessment for each CSS participant. Except for a few variables that refer to past events, all measurements refer to the time of the assessment; therefore, no causality is implied. We have included the nonstatistically significant parameter estimates because these are often of as much interest as the significant estimates.

Although we saw some differences in functioning between age and gender groups, when other variables are included in the analysis, it is clear that by themselves, and on average, age and sex are not significantly related to the level of independence on the Activities of Daily Living. Nor are the race/ethnic indicators or the level of education. Life satisfaction does not seem to be associated significantly with the level of functioning. Living alone or having an episode of bed care because of illness within the two weeks before the assessment are also insignificant. Hearing and vision difficulties appear to have little association with need for help with personal care. The less serious chronic conditions and the proportion of time spent in the hospital in the past six months are also insignificant.

The strongest association, not surprisingly, is between the amount of help the respondent reported needing and the level of ADL functioning. Functioning on the instrumental activities was associated with personal care functioning, as was mental functioning, although to a lesser degree. Walking independently was associated with higher levels of ADL, and those who rated their health as poor were, on average, poorer in functioning in this area. Married persons reported lower ADL functioning, as did those with a larger number of chronic conditions.

The proportion of time an individual spent in a nursing home in the previous six months was associated with a higher level of ADL functioning. This is not unreasonable. We have included in our analyses only the people in the community at the time of assessment. Therefore, anyone assessed who had been in a nursing home had recovered enough function to be discharged.

The analysis explained approximately 43 percent of the variance in ADL level.

Changes in Personal Care Functioning

One area of continuing interest to researchers and planners of programs that serve the elderly is the extent to which functioning changes over time. Many programs include as an objective the maintenance or increase of independence in their clients, yet the underlying suspicion is that the inexorable process of age indicates a natural, if gradual, loss of independent functioning. An additional problem, at least for programs using the ADL as an assessment tool, is that the categories are broad, and are perhaps not fine enough to detect small changes over relatively short periods of time.

Two conditions should be noted here. First, to measure change, the CSS participants had to have at least two assessments, so those who died or refused further participation are not included. Second, an important precondition for change is the initial functioning level. People with high levels of independence have little room for improvement. Conversely, those who are very dependent have little likelihood of getting worse, at least as measured on this scale.

When the individual is a victim of chronic disease, not uncommon in the elderly, significant improvement in functioning may not be likely. Maintenance of existing functioning is a reasonable goal.

A multivariate analysis of the changes in ADL functioning is reported in table 5–4. The dependent variable is the amount of change in ADL functioning in a six-month period. The ADL measurements used to calculate change are those devised by the Multipurpose Senior Services Project in California. Rather than using a simple dichotomous variable to indicate dependence or independence, each item can be rated more finely, making small changes more evident (Lubben 1984). There were only thirty-three individuals who began the period in the low functioning group and were still available for a second assessment.

The variable most strongly associated with change is the original sum of ADL independencies and is very close to one. For example, an original score of six, multiplied by the parameter coefficient would completely offset the intercept of 6.2615, predicting no change in ADL for these people, other conditions being held constant. Males experienced some increase in functioning when other characteristics were held constant. Being black was associated with some decrement, as were the number of chronic diseases, vision difficulties, and the proportion of time in the hospital during the period between the two assessments. Predictably, those who rated their health as poor suffered a decrease in self-care capacity and reporting a need for help was associated with functional loss.

With the exception of gender, all the statistically significant variables were negative. The results of this analysis imply that it is easier to predict decreases in functioning than increases. We turn now to the instrumental activities—those daily chores concerned with maintaining a household, getting places, and managing communications and financial transactions.

Instrumental Activities

Although of a seemingly less critical nature than the ADL tasks, the IADL tasks are necessary to noninstitutional living. Some may not actually be daily tasks (money management or laundry, for example) but all must be performed if a person is to maintain a healthy, safe, and independent life. These

Table 5–4
Results of a regression of various personal characteristics on the change in ADL functioning between the first and second assessments (average six-month period)

Variable	Unstandardized Parameter Estimate	Probability That Estimate Equals 0	Standardized Estimate
(Intercept)	6.2615	0.0001	
Male	0.1212	0.0292	0.0454
Age	−0.0136	0.6705	−0.0094
Original ADL score	−1.0136	0.0001	−1.7067
Life satisfaction	0.0080	0.3836	0.0288
Black	−0.1102	0.0001	−0.0362
Hispanic	−0.0963	0.2212	−0.0256
Other race (nonwhite)	0.0437	0.5413	0.0130
Lives alone	0.0537	0.3787	0.0222
Married	−0.0448	0.5117	−0.0160
Number of serious chronic conditions	−0.1144	0.0678	−0.0369
Number of less serious chronic conditions	0.0055	0.7889	−0.0064
Hearing difficulties	0.0848	0.2554	0.0244
Vision difficulties	−0.1782	0.0078	−0.0578
Amount of informal help	−0.0065	0.5706	−0.0164
Amount of help needed	−0.1103	0.0001	−0.3687
Change in life satisfaction	0.0021	0.7016	0.0101
Proportion of acute care in past six months	−2.5202	0.0001	−0.1055
Proportion of past six months in nursing home	0.2948	0.6073	0.0102
Self-rated health poor	−0.1158	0.0841	−0.0351

Adjusted R^2 = 0.7036, n = 882
Variables whose parameter estimates are significant at p. ≤ 0.10 are in bold.

are also the tasks that are often the first to become difficult for the elderly and disabled to perform. Even the nondisabled may at some point find the heaviest housecleaning activities impossible to perform. Those with disposable income can employ outsiders to help, if family resources are in short supply. The poor must often do without help. They may have to tolerate dingy windows, unvacuumed living space, dirty floors and walls because they cannot do these chores themselves. Short periods of such neglect may be tolerable, but for extended periods, these tasks cannot be omitted without serious consequences to health and hygiene.

Laundry may become impossible, either because there is no laundry equipment available in the living area and the individual can no longer carry the laundry to the nearest laundromat or cleaners, or because of the lack of strength to lift wet wash.

Transportation problems may arise because the individual can no longer drive, or cannot negotiate long walks or the high steps of public transport. Shopping becomes more difficult. Meal preparation depends upon shopping and the manipulation of small tools, which may become difficult for older people stricken with arthritis in their hands or poor vision. Particularly in meal preparation, brain disease or mental illness may make the operation of stoves and other kitchen equipment hazardous.

Cultural mores influence dependency in IADL items. Men in this age group may feel that cooking and cleaning are "women's work" or, if willing, may be ignorant of how to do these tasks. Figure 5–2 data show the distribution of independence on IADL tasks for the CSS participants, presented by sex and age group.

Independence in IADL activities is lower, on average, than ADL independence. Two factors may influence this observation. First, it is likely that individuals expend more effort to maintain their independence in highly personal activities. Second, many of the instrumental activities require more mobility than many elderly can manage. For example, traveling can become hazard-

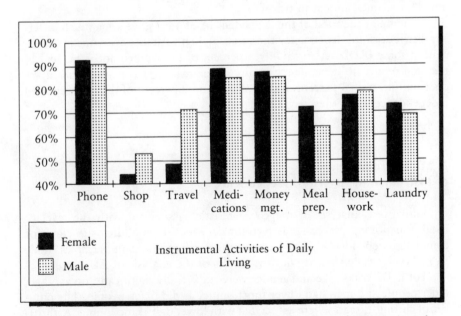

Figure 5–2. Percentage of respondents independent in each Instrumental Activity of Daily Living

ous with limited body strength, particularly for the poor. Taxis are expensive, bus steps are high, a car may not be available, destinations are often too far for walking. Shopping is even more of a problem, as it almost always includes carrying items, often fairly heavy grocery bags.

The highest amount of independence is evident in telephoning; medications and money management are next. These are also the tasks which require the least mobility. Here, men exhibit somewhat more dependence than women. It should be noted here that for the three "domestic" items—food preparation, housework, and laundry—only men who lived alone were evaluated. In many cases, interviewers found that men living with their wives or other female relatives said they could not perform these domestic tasks. These statements were judged to be a result of social role rather than functional limitation. If all men were included, their independence levels would be lower.

Shopping and travel were the areas in which women exhibited the most dependence. As Alice Hughes found, shopping is a major problem for the poor elderly. Without help, they have great difficulty in getting to stores and carrying their purchases. Alice Hughes, despite her crutches, manages much of her traveling by herself. So do a slight majority of the women in this sample. As we saw in chapter 4, those with nearby relatives, unlike Alice Hughes, get much of their help in transportation and shopping from them.

Men show a corresponding problem with shopping; however, they are much more independent in travel.

Looking at the total of the dependent IADL items, we see a much different distribution of dependency than that of ADL. Almost everyone is dependent in some IADL activity. Only 4 percent of the women and 7 percent of the men report no dependency in any of the tasks. At the other end of the distribution, only 3 percent of the women and 2 percent of the men reported independence in all these activities.

A Multivariate Analysis of Instrumental Activity Independence

A multivariate analysis of the characteristics associated with the level of IADL functioning (the range is zero for dependence on all items to eight for complete independence) shows many statistically significant variables (table 5–5). Some are consistent with the results of the analysis of ADL level.

For IADL tasks, age and gender were statistically significant; on average, older people and men had lower functioning, as did black people. The number of chronic diseases were associated with lower daily functioning. Arthritis is a member of the set of conditions. It is frequent in the elderly population

Table 5–5
Results of a regression of various personal characteristics on the sum of independent Instrumental Activities of Daily Living

Variable	Unstandardized Parameter Estimate	Probability That Estimate Equals 0	Standardized Estimate
(Intercept)	4.4645	0.0001	
Aged 85+	−0.1684	0.0256	−0.0426
Male	−0.1550	0.0630	−0.0355
Amount of informal help	−0.0107	0.5034	−0.0178
Sum of ADL items	0.1498	0.0035	0.0673
Sum of correct SPMSQ	0.1299	0.0001	0.1070
Walks independently	0.2419	0.0066	0.0557
Rates health poor	−0.0855	0.4215	−0.0155
Life satisfaction	0.0033	0.6763	0.0076
Black	−0.3646	0.0004	−0.0669
Hispanic	−0.0946	0.4286	−0.0146
Other race (nonwhite)	−0.1262	0.2415	−0.0229
Lives alone	0.4006	0.0001	0.1016
Married	0.1758	0.0887	0.0385
Educational level	0.0696	0.1026	0.0308
In bed in past two weeks	−0.1123	0.2381	−0.0214
Cut activities	0.0353	0.7051	0.0068
Hearing difficulties	−0.0606	0.5706	−0.0108
Vision difficulties	−0.1676	0.4867	−0.0136
Number of serious chronic diseases	−0.1253	0.1713	−0.0252
Number of less serious chronic diseases	−0.0561	0.0696	−0.0400
Proportion of acute care in past six months	−1.0963	0.3174	−0.0178
Proportion of nursing home care in past six months	1.9513	0.0426	−0.0362
Amount of help needed	−0.3020	0.0001	−0.6316

Adjusted R^2 = 0.6971, n = 1328
Variables whose parameter estimates are significant at p. ≤ 0.10 are in bold.

and affects agility and mobility. As with ADL functioning, those who reported needing more help were lower functioning.

There was a positive association between IADL, ADL, and SPMSQ functioning. People tend to have general levels of good or poor functioning, affecting all areas of their lives. Those who walk independently quite naturally function better in daily life, and both the married and those who live alone function better. Once again, those who were in a nursing home in the past six months had, on average, better functioning than others like them who were not institutionalized.

The nonsignificant estimates tell part of the story, also. The amount of informal help one was receiving was not associated with IADL functioning as it was with personal care functioning. Those who rated their health as poor were, on average, functioning the same as their counterparts in these areas. Many of the estimates of the parameters for the health characteristics were insignificant.

On the whole, although the analysis explained almost 70 percent of the variance in IADL level, only the amount of help needed was a substantively significant influence on instrumental activity capacity of the respondents.

Changes in Instrumental Activity Functioning

Changes in IADL independence are likely to be more evident over time than those of ADL items. Individuals are more apt to struggle to maintain their independence in personal care items, but be less sensitive about receiving help with household chores. Intuitively, we would probably all feel much more dependent if we had to request help in dressing ourselves or bathing than if we needed help with heavy housecleaning.

There was much more change evident in IADL dependence than in the previously discussed ADL dependence. Most of the variance in changes in IADL functioning can be explained by a number of characteristics measured in the assessment or from medical records. Table 5–6 data show the results of a regression of these characteristics on change in IADL functioning between the first and second assessments.

Just as with ADL, the original IADL score had the most influence in predicting possible change over the six-month period. Older people had more loss than younger people. Those persons who were Asian, American Indian, or Filipino were more likely to have reduced capacity at the second assessment. The more chronic conditions, the more likely a loss. Both the amount of help one received and the amount that was needed were associated with IADL functioning change. Those who rated their health as poor and those who had had a recent nursing home stay were more likely to have a decrease in functioning.

Only the parameters for being married or living alone had positive, statistically significant estimates.

Mental Status

Senility is the popular term for the often expected loss of mental acuity presumed to accompany aging. Whatever the incidence, and whatever the causes, poor mental functioning has serious ramifications for independent living. Individuals who otherwise enjoy good health and who are physically

Table 5–6
Results of a regression of various personal characteristics on the change
in IADL functioning between the first and second assessments
(average six-month period)

Variable	Unstandardized Parameter Estimate	Probability That Estimate Equals 0	Standardized Estimate
(Intercept)	9.2352	0.0001	
Male	−0.0974	0.2589	−0.0151
Age	−0.0236	0.0001	−0.0589
Original IADL score	−1.0241	0.0001	−0.7260
Life satisfaction	0.0017	0.8806	0.0026
Black	−0.0535	0.5845	−0.0073
Hispanic	−0.0320	0.7925	−0.0036
Other race (nonwhite)	−0.2602	0.0199	−0.0322
Lives alone	0.3184	0.0009	0.0546
Married	0.1750	0.0991	0.0260
Number of serious chronic conditions	−0.1906	0.0493	−0.0258
Number of less serious chronic conditions	−0.0690	0.0305	−0.0333
Hearing difficulties	0.0424	0.7166	0.0050
Vision difficulties	0.0535	0.6064	0.0072
Amount of informal help	−0.0547	0.0025	−0.0572
Amount of help needed	−0.3612	0.0001	−0.4988
Change in life satisfaction	0.0004	0.9663	0.0007
Proportion of acute care in past six months	−0.5927	0.4681	−0.0092
Proportion of past six months in nursing home	−1.7863	0.0469	−0.0251
Self-rated health poor	−0.2787	0.0076	−0.0352

Adjusted $R^2 = 0.8801$, n $= 882$
Variables whose parameter estimates are significant at p. ≤ 0.10 are in bold.

capable of performing all the daily activities, may be completely dependent because they lack judgment about when and how to do what needs to be done to maintain themselves.

For people who need twenty-four-hour supervision, the probability of home care is limited. Programs that might meet this kind of need have limited funding; families provide much of the help, but often at great physical and emotional cost to the caregiver. While there are many measures of emotional and mental illness, the measure we report is one often used to determine the mental acuity of the elderly population. It is intended to test the respondent's orientation in time and the short-term memory.

The Short Portable Mental Status Questionnaire is intended to measure the possible presence or absence of organic brain disease. The following questions are asked of the respondent:

1. "What day of the week is it?"
2. "What is the date today?"
3. "Who is the president of the United States now?"
4. "Who was the president just before him?"
5. "Subtract three from twenty and keep subtracting three from each number, all the way down."
6. "What is your telephone number?" (If the respondent has no telephone, street address is substituted.)
7. "What is the name of this place?"
8. "How old are you?"
9. "When were you born?"
10. "What is your mother's maiden name?"

For the California Senior Survey, as is often done in surveys which include people of all races and educational backgrounds, adjustments were made for those variables. A commonly used categorization places respondents in categories based on the number of incorrect answers: intact, mild impairment, moderate impairment, or severe impairment. The scores are relative, placing respondents upon a continuum.

Our sample showed little brain disease, at least as measured by the SPMSQ. The distribution is not unlike the distribution of ADL independence. The great majority of the respondents show no impairment in orientation and memory. When those with mild impairment are included, more than 95 percent of the sample have few problems in this area (see table 5–7).

Table 5–7

Percentage distribution of number of incorrect responses to the SPMSQ

Number of Incorrect Responses	Category	Female %	Male %
8–10	Severe	1.02	0.48
5–7	Moderate	4.73	2.90
3–4	Mild	12.25	9.93
0–2	Intact	82.00	86.68

A Multivariate Analysis of Mental Functioning

A more interesting way to examine the differences between the respondents and their level of mental functioning is to regress a set of personal characteristics on the total number of correct responses to the questionnaire. How much help in judging an individual's mental acuity can be gained by knowing about other facets of his or her life? Table 5–8 data show the results of a multivariate regression of these characteristics on the number of correct answers.

Table 5–8
Results of a regression of various personal characteristics on the sum of correct responses to Short Portable Mental Status Questionnaire

Variable	Unstandardized Parameter Estimate	Probability That Estimate Equals 0	Standardized Estimate
(Intercept)	6.3952	0.0001	
Aged 85 +	−0.2086	0.0364	−0.0641
Male	0.2464	0.0253	0.0685
Amount of informal help	−0.0215	0.3063	−0.0437
Sum of ADL items	0.1482	0.0291	−0.0808
Sum of IADL items	0.2269	0.0001	−0.2754
Walks independently	−0.1842	0.1183	−0.0515
Rates health poor	0.0366	0.7944	0.0081
Life satisfaction	0.0146	0.1566	0.0412
Black	0.3441	0.0117	0.0766
Hispanic	0.3072	0.0517	0.0576
Other race (nonwhite)	−0.1663	0.2433	−0.0366
Lives alone	0.2881	0.0182	0.0887
Married	0.5265	0.0001	0.1401
Educational level	−0.1098	0.0515	−0.0589
In bed in past two weeks	−0.0196	0.8760	−0.0045
Cut activities	0.2718	0.0274	0.0635
Hearing difficulties	−0.2253	0.1105	−0.0485
Vision difficulties	−0.4050	0.0016	−0.0992
Number of serious chronic diseases	0.0447	0.7119	−0.0109
Number of less serious chronic diseases	0.1760	0.0001	0.1522
Proportion of acute care in past six months	1.1617	0.2645	0.0318
Proportion of nursing home care in past six months	1.7478	0.1697	0.0393
Amount of help needed	−0.0231	0.3342	−0.0586

Adjusted R^2 = 0.2205, n = 1328
Variables whose parameter estimates are significant at p. ≤ 0.10 are in bold.

The personal characteristics associated with mental functioning as measured by the SPMSQ are numerous, but the entire set explain only 22 percent of the variance in the sum of correct answers. The following variables are associated with lower scores: being eighty-five years old or older (lending credence to our suspicion that mental problems accompany old age) and suffering visual difficulties. Men, on average, tended toward a higher score. Race, ethnicity, and educational level were statistically significant, but no doubt more a result of the adjustments made to the scale than any inherent difference. Being married, living alone, or having curtailed activities during the two weeks prior to the assessment were also associated with higher SPMsQ levels. Higher numbers of chronic diseases were also associated, but may merely indicate that those with better memory could report more problems.

As one would guess from the analyses of ADL and IADL functioning, SPMSQ functioning is positively associated with those scales.

Changes in SPMSQ Functioning

Changes in mental functioning are somewhat more difficult to assess. Common sense would dictate the belief that in a six-month period, the most likely result would be maintenance of mental acuity. However, the CSS participants, at least those in the medium group, showed more improvement than would be expected. Thirty-three percent of the women and 42 percent of the men in that group showed improvement.

As we look at the questions, we wonder what degree of learning may have taken place. For example, of all the people who could not remember who the last president was or remember their mother's maiden name, at least some of them would be expected to think about it and perhaps be prepared for the question next time around. Therefore, to assess mental functioning change, we arbitrarily designated a change as a change of more than two in either direction to qualify as significant mental functioning change.

A regression of characteristics on the change in mental functioning explained 64 percent variance in that measure, although only a few of the variables were statistically significant. Table 5-9 presents the parameter estimates resulting from a regression of personal characteristics on the change in mental functioning.

Consistent with the earlier analysis, increasing age is associated with decreasing mental acuity. The SPMSQ grouping at the first assessment was the strongest predictor of change, just as the original groupings in the ADL and IADL analyses were the most important predictors. Life satisfaction, not surprisingly, was associated with improvement, as was living alone or being married. But change in the level of life satisfaction was not significantly asso-

Table 5–9
Results of a regression of various personal characteristics on the change in SPMSQ functioning between the first and second assessments (average six-month period)

Variable	Unstandardized Parameter Estimate	Probability That Estimate Equals 0	Standardized Estimate
(Intercept)	10.3733	0.0001	
Male	0.0920	0.4528	0.0172
Age	−0.0190	0.0185	−0.0574
Original SPMSQ score	−1.0813	0.0001	−0.7376
Life satisfaction	0.0350	0.0333	0.0630
Black	0.3592	0.0099	0.0590
Hispanic	0.4723	0.0068	0.0627
Other race (nonwhite)	0.2206	0.1628	0.0327
Lives alone	0.2669	0.0478	0.0552
Married	0.4002	0.0081	0.0714
Number of serious chronic conditions	0.1358	0.3262	0.0219
Number of less serious chronic conditions	0.1185	0.0093	0.0686
Hearing difficulties	−0.3696	0.0250	−0.0531
Vision difficulties	0.1237	0.4025	0.0201
Amount of informal help	0.0096	0.7038	0.0121
Amount of help needed	−0.1518	0.0001	−0.2538
Change in life satisfaction	−0.0181	0.1294	−0.0444
Proportion of acute care in past six months	−1.1526	0.2679	−0.0241
Proportion of past six months in nursing home	0.6645	0.5975	0.1147
Self-rated health poor	0.0864	0.5592	0.0131

Adjusted $R^2 = 0.6381$, n = 882
Variables whose parameter estimate are significant at p. ≤ 0.10 are in bold.

ciated with change in mental functioning. Just as in the other analyses of functioning, needing higher amounts of help was associated with loss of function, as was poor hearing. Once again, race, ethnicity, and educational level (all adjustments to the score) were significant. However, we would expect the effect to remain constant, since the adjustments would be the same for both administrations of the questionnaire.

The analysis explained 64 percent of the variance in mental functioning change, and probably most of that is attributable to knowing the original SPMSQ group to which individuals belonged.

Summary

The most general summarizing statement about functioning is that functioning in all areas of living for the poor elderly tend to be of the same general relative level. A person who is independent in the instrumental activities of daily living is highly likely to be independent in personal care and in mental functioning. The reverse is not quite as certain. Because of the personal nature of the ADL items, individuals, through modesty or a desire to avoid the intimacy with another person that necessarily accompanies such care, may struggle harder to maintain independence in these areas.

Change in the three areas also tends to occur in the same direction. When a person is suffering a loss of self-care capacity, usually it is not confined to just one area of life; all parts may suffer.

The most telling variable in the analysis of change was the original level of functioning. That is, at least in the short term, if one knows how well a person is functioning, one can make, on average, an informed judgment about future functioning. The most difficulty would come in predicting a person's future IADL functioning. Here, stability is not the rule as in the other two indices.

If we were to apply the generalized indications of functional change to the individual case of Alice Hughes, we would expect her to maintain her mental functioning and the high degree of personal care capacity she exhibits. We would be less likely to believe that her ability to perform the instrumental activities of daily living will stay the same. Her functioning falls into the middle group of IADL functioning, so the expectation would be for some change in either direction.

6
Care and Its Cost

Allie Minships

Allie Minships calls herself "the walker," but it is amazing that she can function at all. She has endured eight operations: four for gallstones, one on her knee, two for cataracts, and one on her neck. She has seven collapsed vertebrae; bone has been removed from her right hip to support her neck and she is in constant pain. She wears a neck collar and special shoes for a heel spur (lump) on her right foot. Apparently, she has a rare bone disease discovered while she lived in Florida. Allie Minships has the dubious distinction of being among three in Florida stricken with the malady, identified as Pagents Disease.

Allie has had contact with many, if not most, of the medical care providers in San Franciso—St. Francis Hospital, Pacific Presbyterian Medical Center, the podiatry medical school, and its clinic.

Today, Allie is a member of the Healthwise Senior Plan of St. Francis Hospital. She is free of medications, even though she daily manages emphysema, angina, an ulcer, a hernia of the stomach (which forces her to sleep sitting up), and chronic neck pain.

Allie was born in New York City in 1903. She is eighty-four and appears decades younger. She remembers being sickly most of her life. Today, however, this tiny Caucasian woman with wild, curly brown hair sparkles with energy.

She has lived on the edge of poverty all her life. Her mother took in washing and her father worked as a waiter around the tenements of the city. Allie used to pick up dropped leftover coal from the coal trains on Riverside Drive.

Allie remembers being hungry a lot of the time. When she was ten years old, she worked in a grocery store delivering milk. She had completed one year of high school when her mother died; Allie was sixteen years old.

Her mother's death marked a dark time in Allie's life. She was sent away to live with an aunt, then to a friend, then to another friend, then kicked out of still another home. She had no place to live and her father did not care for her. Allie lost contact with her brother and was able to survive by washing dishes in boarding houses and caring for babies.

Her misfortune continued when she married a Russian cemetery gardener in 1923 and gave birth to a daughter. Her husband beat her and later left her alone to bear a son. During the marriage, Allie developed a heart condition and left her husband in 1928. Neither remarried. He died twenty-five years ago. Today, the daughter is sixty-one and the son fifty-eight, and Allie's relationship with them is distant and poor. She knows she has eleven grandchildren and that her daughter was widowed, but little else.

Allie's current life in a small room in a Tenderloin hotel in San Francisco came by way of a move to Florida. At her son-in-law's invitation, Allie followed her daughter's family when the son-in-law's ship was reassigned from Brooklyn Navy Yard to Florida. She resided there for twenty-seven years, and her relationship with her family deteriorated.

Looking back now, Allie reflects that "Florida was a trap." She was living in the Royal Motel and trading labor as a gardener for free rent for a cottage. When Allie was sixty-nine, the landlady sold the motel and Allie's future looked grim.

She decided to make a desperate move and grasp at a long-held dream to live in San Francisco. She had seventy-five dollars in life savings, but a one-way bus ticket to San Francisco was ninety-five dollars. Allie borrowed twenty dollars from her landlady and arrived in San Francisco on Ash Wednesday in 1973. She had no money and it was her seventieth birthday.

Again reflecting, Allie muses that she "did everything right, ya know." She followed the dictates for women of her youth. She worked hard most of her life. Before World War II she enjoyed a respectable job as a clerk bookkeeper for a Wall Street insurance company. During the war she worked for Brooklyn Western Electric as a drill press operator, manufacturing needles.

The soiled broken plaster walls in Allie's room are covered with pennants and pictures of life in San Francisco. She sleeps on a single day bed. The room also contains a chair, a dresser with broken knobs, a mini-refrigerator, a miniature desk, and a small television. Somewhere behind a drape that covers a bookshelf is a hot plate.

Allie's limited energy is dedicated to community service. She is excited by the challenge and enjoys her work. Her public involvement began in the mid-1970s when she became a page at KQED, a public television station. She worked her way up to the position of head page and met a lot of popular entertainers.

During 1978 and 1979 Allie attracted a brief fame when she was written up in the 13 May 1979 Datebook, "Profiles of Four Inspired Women." The article describes Allie's trials and her courage. Almost ten years later the cut-out article is brown and soiled and hanging by torn duct tape on her wall.

Allie also has been a pillar of the Downtown Senior Center across the street from her hotel for thirteen years. She is an active member of the rhythm band and enjoys the close friendship of the three other women in the band. They spend time together shopping, cooking, and entertaining at convalescent hospitals and for the Shriners. Allie has a photograph of "the girls" dressed in bright 1920s outfits.

When Allie is not working with the band she crochets clothing sets for babies and children for community bazaars. She sews constantly and simply follows pattern books. She makes some for the Fire Department service to poor Asian children. She also sews for Raphael House, for the homeless. Allie would crochet and donate much more, but the wool yarn is expensive.

Ill health followed Allie Minships into her eighth decade. She still walks to the hospital, but takes a senior van home. Nowadays, Medi-Cal covers most of her health care costs, which have been considerable. Allie reports "beautiful care" and "gorgeous food" while hospitalized for her various surgeries. Before Medi-Cal, most of her hospital experiences were "charity cases." A major surgery was paid for by the Elks Club. Allie does not wish to be hospitalized. When she had neck surgery she was an inpatient for eleven days. "I begged them to go home all the time; I feel safe here in the hotel."

Allie has never received In-Home Supportive Services but several years ago she received services at the Department of Public Health Central City Senior's Unit. Allie reports that "the community mental health services may have helped me in the beginning, but today she (the worker) is useless. I think she has her own set of problems." Allie is finding it difficult to disentangle herself from the mental health worker. "She calls and bothers me all the time." The worker called during this interview and Allie firmly declined intervention.

Allie wishes to spend the remainder of her life paying back to the community the good she has received. Allie stares at the wall covered by souvenirs and explains that one is really by one's self, and there is another secret story about her life she does not care to reveal. Brushing that aside, it is time to dash off to band practice at the senior center. Words—"I could not live without the center"—trail down the dingy hall as Allie dashes off to the elevator.

The Continuum of Care

Our previous chapters have discussed the degrees of dependency among the old and poor and varying use of formal services. Gertrude Aston fights to maintain her independence; she keeps from her daughter information about a recent fall. An In-Home Supportive Services chore provider comes five days a week to help with the housework and Gertrude's family maintains close contact. Her health is relatively good, but she takes medication for her chronic heart and blood pressure problems.

Agnes Hughes, on the other hand, has no family available. A chore provider from a private agency, paid for by the IHSS program, comes twice a week to clean the house and purchase groceries. Agnes has had surgery annually for the past few years, once for bowel problems and the rest for hip problems and replacements. Her hip problems make it precarious for her to bath alone; getting in and out of the tub is difficult. The chore provider helps with her bath and domestic chores.

Iris Carlton, in relatively good health and with no recent surgeries, receives help from her family and church friends. So far she has not needed help from public agencies, except for a bus "Fast Pass."

Judy Anderson, like Agnes Hughes, has a history of hip surgeries and replacements and has a chore worker to help with housework. She, too, suffered a fall, which resulted in a broken arm. Three of these four women, although selected randomly on the basis of other characteristics, receive help in their homes provided through public programs, help that permits them to maintain their independence.

As we saw in chapter 5 and in the brief descriptions of the functioning of the women, dependency moves along a continuum. Some individuals are quite independent, needing very little outside help to maintain themselves and carry out their domestic and personal chores. Others, fewer than we might have expected, need all help possible to maintain themselves. Most fall somewhere between, either as a result of the deterioration of physical functioning associated with old age and chronic illness, or as the result of acute medical conditions that severely limit their ability to care for themselves and their surroundings.

The continuum of care concept refers to the health and social services that meet the needs of people at particular points in a continuum of dependency. At one end are those who are ambulatory and usually independent; at the other end are those who need twenty-four-hour care to live safely (Minkler and Blum 1982). The range of services along the continuum can be from services as noncritical and intermittent as information and referral to those as intense and skilled as acute care in a hospital.

In the first two sections of this chapter we separate the social and medical services. In the last section we look at experiences of the CSS sample that take into account not only the amount of social and medical services, but the movement of the individuals between community and institutional care. Popular expositions on the problems of aging tend to concentrate on hospital and nursing home care, financially the most obvious cost of caring for the old and poor.

Public policy in services for the elderly is an example of the paradox between popular belief and the manifest ends of service funding. Rhetoric surrounding the care of the dependent elderly decries the notion of nursing home care, except in the most extreme cases. Institutionalization is bad; maintaining independence in the community is good.

However, the primary funding sources for services for the elderly and poor—Medicare and Medicaid—provide incentives for institutionalization (Kane and Kane 1980). Neither program, except in special circumstances, provides for services in the home, particularly if they are not planned and approved by a physician. However, increasing costs for hospitalization and nursing home care have forced changes on both systems.

Social Services

The most general problems of social services have been coordination, accessibility, and availability. Providing services in the community, unlike medical services in institutions, means making services known to people in the community, being able to meet the very diverse needs of a group with a wide range of disability, and being able to provide the needed services. In many communities, it is relatively easy to obtain domestic services for those who can no longer do heavy housework. It is much more difficult, almost everywhere, to provide the respite care needed, for example, for those caretakers of individuals suffering from the debilitation of Alzheimer's disease.

Services for the elderly are provided through public, nonprofit, and for-profit service organizations. In the public sector, the programs most likely to fund services for the elderly are Title XX (now known as the Social Service Block Grant) of the Social Security Act and the Older Americans Act, passed in 1965. Part of the mandate of the Older Americans Act was to serve as an agency responsible for planning and coordination of services. However, limited funding and limited authority over the many service agencies has diluted the intent of the act (Estes 1979).

Because of the relative size of the expenditures and the rapid inflation in the cost of service, medical services tend to be in the spotlight in any discussion of services for the elderly. However, this decade has seen a surge of interest in community care, so that the provision of social services in the community has attained more prominence. This interest is based on the hope that providing services to clients in their homes will permit them to remain independent. They will presumably not be forced to enter nursing homes for primarily nonmedical problems—the inability to maintain themselves and their surroundings.

Table 6–1 shows the distribution of the number of services received by each CSS participant. Almost 67 percent of the participants reported receiving *no* services and it is well to remember that in this chapter we are talking about formal services only. Persons receiving no formal services are not nec-

Table 6–1
Distribution of number of formal services received at first assessment

Number of services	Number of recipients	%
None	879	66.9
One	275	21.0
Two	103	7.9
Three	39	3.0
Four	9	0.6
Five	4	0.3
Six	1	0.1
Seven	2	0.2

essarily demonstrating lack of need for services. They may be receiving help from family, friends, or neighbors. In some cases, but not identified here, they may need the help, but it isn't available in their community. Or, while an observer might conclude that a person needs help, he or she (preferring not to appear dependent) may report "getting along just fine."

Another 29 percent receive only one or two services, and very few receive more than two services—slightly over 4 percent. Although there are many types of services that may be presumed to be needed by the old and poor, it appears that most individuals actually avail themselves of only one or two services. Reasons for not using services include personal independence, lack of awareness of services available, family help, or services not available.

Table 6–2 provides a more specific look at the types of services used and the predominant provider agency for the services used by this group. If we apply the notion of a continuum of care with respect to social services, we can see that many of these services are at the lower end. They are available to individuals whose need for help is limited or perhaps confined to one particular area. Some, like legal assistance, are not necessarily dependent upon independence in self-maintenance but upon the unavailability of certain expensive professional services to those with few resources.

Others are more clearly tied to the notion of independence or dependence. A person who can quite competently provide for her own domestic and personal care may still need transportation for medical appointments and shopping. A person's dependence may be caused by mental or physical problems; protective services are a response to the potential of abuse or neglect because of a person's mental incapacity to protect herself.

Table 6–2 data show the distribution of *services* received; some recipients received more than one service. For the one-third of the participants who received any formal services, the average number of services received was 1.6. These figures represent the response to the service questions at the first assessment. They are the number of services received at a particular time, not the number of services received over a time period.

Table 6–2
Number of percentage of formal services received, by provider agency type, at first assessment

Service Group	Number	% of Total	Number by Provider Agency A	B	C	D*
Adult social day care	20	2.93	9	10	1	0
Housing (education, minor repair, emergency shelter)	34	4.97	12	20	2	0
IHSS (chore, personal care, health or meal related)	268	49.25	207	28	28	5
Legal (representation, assistance)	14	2.05	9	2	3	0
Respite (in- or out-of-home)	8	1.17	0	2	3	0
Nonmedical transportation (regular, specially equipped, escort)	120	17.57	57	47	11	5
Meals (congregate, home-delivered)	50	7.32	7	36	6	1
Protective services (money mgt., guardianship, telephone reassurance, visiting)	18	2.64	8	6	2	2
Special communication (translation, devices)	5	0.73	3	1	1	0
Preventive health care	11	1.61	5	0	6	0
Senior center attendance (with or without meal)	135	19.77	63	60	2	10

*A = Public, B = Nonprofit, C = Private/Profit, D = Unknown

Almost half the services used fall into the in-home services category. This is not surprising, as California has an extensive, statewide In-Home Supportive Services program, funded through Title XX, available to the elderly disabled SS/SSP recipients. Providers of these services do as little as once-a-year heavy housecleaning or occasional wintertime snow removal to as much as daily domestic and personal care. Clients are assessed by a county IHSS caseworker and allotted a certain number of hours monthly for the services they need. There are statewide guidelines, primarily describing the maximum hours that can be awarded and distinguishing between nonseverely and severely impaired persons. Counties form their own guidelines as to how many hours are awarded and often set maxima for particular sets of services, such as domestic, meals, and personal care.

This service is obviously quite important in the prevention of unnecessary institutionalization. Although the program has never analyzed the actual incidence of institutionalization, nor does it have comparative figures for individuals receiving IHSS and not receiving it, political rhetoric surrounding the program is usually based on the assumption that it does, in fact, prevent nursing home use. At the time of this survey, the IHSS program served approximately 10 percent of the state SSI/SSP recipient population.

The second-most-used service is senior center attendance. This service can be somewhat interdependent with IHSS for severely disabled elders, as while they are at the senior center, they don't need personal care in their homes. Senior center attendance is highly dependent upon the availability of such centers. California's Adult Day Health Care program, now expanding, was actually only available in three of the areas in which CSS participants lived.

Transportation services are an obvious need for the elderly, poor or not. Public transportation is often unavailable, and those afflicted with certain types of chronic disease, such as arthritis, may not be able to get on and off buses.

Nutrition is often a problem for the elderly. Aside from any financial or transportational difficulties in attaining a variety of foods, the elderly, particularly those without family, can suffer from isolation resulting in less motivation to prepare meals and eat. Others suffer disabilities that make cooking dangerous. Meal services are provided in three of the service categories. An IHSS worker may prepare meals for a client, meals can be furnished at senior centers, or prepared meals can be delivered by agencies such as Meals-on-Wheels. Senior centers may provide a nutritious hot meal as part of their program.

Interviewers also ascertained the type of provider agency for the services respondents reported receiving. Fifty-six percent of the services were provided by public agencies and another 31 percent were provided by private, nonprofit agencies. Private, for-profit agencies accounted for 10 percent of the services provided. In 3 percent of the reported services, the agency status was unknown.

Only in the respite care and preventive health care categories were for-profit agencies the predominant providers, and these are among the categories with the smallest representation.

Are there significant differences in service use by age? We saw in chapter 5 that dependency is related to age; on average, it increases with advancing age and we might expect that service use would reflect that association. Table 6–3 data provide a look at the service use of the participants in each age group. For example, 7.5 percent of those in the lowest age group, sixty-five to seventy-four, use housing services, while only 2.4 percent of the oldest (eighty-five and older) report using housing services.

The differences for the most part are not significant, but some categories do reflect the correspondence between the continuums of dependence and care and their relationship with increasing age. The use of IHSS services increases with age, while the use of nonmedical transportation and senior center services seems to decrease. This is reasonable, since the use of the latter two services implies at least enough independence to leave the home, to have some mobility. Aging is associated with decreased mobility.

Table 6–3
Percentage of CSS participants in age group categories receiving formal services, at first assessment, by service category

	Age Categories		
Percentage of recipients:	*65–74 years*	*75–84 years*	*85 years +*
	41%	*40%*	*19%*
Service	*%*	*%*	*%*
Adult social day care	3.6	2.6	2.4
Housing services	7.5	3.7	2.4
IHSS services	35.8	38.2	49.0
Legal services	2.5	1.9	1.6
Respite care	1.1	0.7	2.4
Nonmedical transportation	13.3	22.2	17.6
Meals (non-IHSS)	8.2	7.0	5.6
Protective services	2.9	1.5	4.8
Communication services	0.4	1.5	0.0
Preventive health services	1.4	1.9	1.6
Senior center services	23.3	18.9	13.6

Table 6–4 data show the distribution of recipients of formal services by racial/ethnic categories. There are some differences, which may be explained by the environment or particular program policies. For example, blacks are more apt to use housing services, reflecting the past emphasis in housing to provide for the most disadvantaged. Fewer Spanish participants reported using IHSS services, but this may be offset by the higher proportion reporting

Table 6–4
Percentage of CSS participants in major racial/ethnic categories receiving formal services, at first assessment, by service category

	Racial/Ethnic Categories			
Percentage of recipients:	*White*	*Black*	*Spanish*	*Asian*
	61%	*26%*	*9%*	*4%*
Service	*%*	*%*	*%*	*%*
Adult social day care	2.4	4.3	3.5	0.0
Housing services	3.2	10.4	5.3	4.6
IHSS services	40.4	41.5	29.8	45.5
Legal services	2.6	2.4	0.0	0.0
Respite care	1.6	0.0	1.8	0.0
Nonmedical transportation	17.4	17.7	17.5	22.7
Meals (non-IHSS)	7.9	4.3	5.3	18.2
Protective services	3.4	1.2	3.5	0.0
Communication services	0.5	0.6	0.0	4.6
Preventive health services	1.9	1.2	1.8	0.0
Senior center services	18.7	16.5	31.6	4.6

the use of senior centers. The small proportion of Asians reported more non-IHSS-provided meals and more communication services.

Table 6–5 data show the results of a regression analysis of the determinants of the number of formal services (including none) used by CSS participants at the time of their first assessment. This particular assessment was chosen to show what services from the existing system were being used by these elderly Medi-Cal recipients. Later assessments were not very different, but there is always the risk that the results could have been contaminated by information about services from the interviewer. Or, answering all the questions about services might provide information new to the respondent.

The results showed that while many variables were associated with the number of formal services, the effect of each by itself was, in most cases, quite small. As expected, the higher a person's independence in the Activities of Daily Living, the Instrumental Activities of Daily Living, and walking, the fewer formal services received, on average.

Interestingly, the higher the educational level and the higher the mental capacity, the higher the number of services. This result reflects the notion

Table 6–5
Determinants of number of formal services received at time of first assessment

Variable	Parameter Estimate	Standard Error	Probability Estimate Is Significant
(Intercept)	0.2832	0.4600	0.5382
ADL independence	−0.0670	0.0394	0.0898
Age (65–100+)	0.0084	0.0039	0.0323
Alone (1 if yes)	0.4004	0.0668	0.0001
Black (1 if yes)	0.2633	0.0711	0.0002
Chronic conditions 1(1–4)	0.0875	0.0630	0.1651
Chronic conditions 2	0.0582	0.0235	0.0132
Education level (1–4)	0.0746	0.0307	0.0153
Poor hearing (1 if yes)	−0.1540	0.0811	0.0580
IADL independence	−0.3110	0.0626	0.0001
Inbed (1 if yes)	−0.0251	0.0702	0.7204
Impaired judgement (1 if yes)	−0.0045	0.0324	0.8896
Married (1 if yes)	0.1807	0.0744	0.0153
MSQ independence	0.0343	0.0187	0.0663
Informal support strength	−0.0614	0.0101	0.0001
Sex (1 if male)	−0.0676	0.0600	0.2599
Spanish (1 if yes)	0.1326	0.0890	0.1364
Asian (1 if yes)	−0.0903	0.0987	0.3606
Self-rated health (1–3)	0.0261	0.0418	0.5327
Poor vision (1 if yes)	−0.0628	0.0723	0.3848
Independent in walking (1 if yes)	−0.1534	0.0663	0.0208

Note: Variables whose estimates are statistically significant at p < .10 are in bold face.
$R^2 = 0.1604$

that people may need a certain level of awareness and ability to find and secure services from the many agencies and programs that do exist. Living alone, being older, and being black all predicted higher formal service use, although the effects are relatively small.

Not surprisingly, the more informal help a person receives, the fewer formal services they are apt to use.

Costs of services received by the CSS participants was particularly hard to ascertain, given the nature of such services. For those who are receiving services funded through public programs, the actual cost of the service is often not known. In the course of evaluating California's MSSP program, the average monthly cost for the reported formal services was calculated for the CSS participants for fiscal year 1980–81 and is presented in table 6–6.

The total cost per month, on average, for CSS participants during this time period was $91.93 (including those who used no services).

More than 60 percent of the average cost of formal services per month is composed of IHSS services. These services, provided in one form or another in all fifty states, provide help with the tasks of everyday living that become more and more onerous for those afflicted with chronic disease. The other major expenditure was for public housing or rent subsidies.

Table 6–6
Average monthly cost of formal services received, by service category, 1980–81

Service Group	Average Cost per Month	Percentage of Monthly Cost
Adult social day care	$ 3.60	3.9
Housing (education, minor repair, emergency shelter)	0.07	0.1
IHSS (chore, personal care, health or meal related)	56.17	61.1
Legal (representation, assistance)	0.23	0.3
Respite (In- or out-of-home)	0.10	0.1
Nonmedical transportation (regular, specially equipped, escort)	1.04	1.1
Meals (congregate, home-delivered)	1.70	1.8
Protective services (money mgt., guardianship, telephone reassurance, visiting)	0.40	0.4
Special communication (translation, devices)	0.03	<0.1
Preventive health care	0.06	0.1
Senior center attendance (with or without meal)	0.15	0.2
Public housing or rent subsidies	20.84	22.6
Other	7.56	8.2
Total Average Cost per Month	$91.93	100.0%

Adapted from Miller, Robert H. "Preliminary Report on the Prices of Referred Services."

Medical Services

Medical services and costs reflect the two specters of old age—increasing medical problems and the rapidly increasing costs of those services during the past two decades. With the attenuation of death by the historical killers of the old and weak—pneumonia and influenza—the elderly live longer, and in so doing, become prey to chronic diseases which, while not immediately fatal, often entail costly and continuing medical care. Even with medical insurance, the cost of medical services to treat those conditions has risen rapidly, outdistancing the ability of elders on a fixed income to pay for the care.

In 1965, Title XVIII of the Social Security Act created the Medicare program—a federal insurance program that helps pay for medical care of the elderly. This program, while containing several coinsurance features and not covering some of the needs of the elderly, provides for their major acute care needs. It is composed of two parts, A and B.

Eligibility for part A, the Hospital Insurance (HI) plan, is linked to the Social Security Retirement Benefits, making eligibility available to almost everyone sixty-five and older. The 1972 amendments to Title XVIII permitted those ineligible to participate to HI. People were ineligible either because they did not meet employment criteria or did not fall under certain transitional rules promulgated at the start of Medicare. Such people were permitted to voluntarily enroll in the program through payment of monthly premiums.

Part A covers inpatient services such as room and meals, nursing services, drugs provided while the patient is in the hospital, medical social services, and supplies and equipment in the hospital. A beneficiary is entitled to a certain number of days of service in a benefit period, and also has a number of lifetime reserve days that can be used in case of very long inpatient stays. Part A also covers one hundred days of skilled nursing care following a hospital stay of at least three days.

Part B, the Supplementary Medical Insurance (SMI) program, is theoretically available to all people sixty-five and older, even if they do not qualify for HI (Davidson and Marmor 1980). Therefore, all aged are eligible for Medicare benefits, given that they either qualify under the Social Security Law or elect to pay premiums voluntarily.

Services provided under Part B are physician services, outpatient hospital care, ambulance services, physical therapy, speech therapy, diagnostic tests, prosthetic devices, and various other services. Prescription drugs are not covered, nor are many home-based services suitable for those who are chronically ill but need not be hospitalized.

While Medicare covers many services, the combination of premiums, deductibles, and copayments combine to form too large an outlay for many elderly persons. The program that helps to fill that gap for the poor is Medicaid.

Medicaid is the state-administered medical benefits program for people below the poverty income, funded by the states and Title XIX of the Social Security Amendments. Eligibility is linked to the cash assistance programs—the primary program for this group of elderly is SSI.

Medicaid is a state program funded jointly with the federal government. States are given much discretion over the services that may be provided under the program. Services that must be provided (including only those applicable to the aged) are inpatient and outpatient hospital services, X-ray and laboratory services, physicians' services, and skilled nursing services. Transportation to and from medical services must be provided, if needed. States may elect to provide additional services. California, the state of residence of the CSS sample, also provides optometry service, podiatrist visits, chiropractic services, dental services, physical therapy, eyeglasses, prescription drugs, prosthetic devices, emergency hospital services, intermediate care, inpatient hospital care for the elderly mentally ill, and other diagnostic, screening, and rehabilitation services.

For the old and poor, Medicare and Medicaid benefits are coordinated by a "buy-in" agreement. This agreement permits the state Medicaid program to pay the premiums, the deductible and coinsurance amounts of those services covered by Medicare. This creates crossover claims for which Medicare pays its benefits and Medicaid pays the remainder. Without this agreement, the shared-cost feature of Medicare would be beyond the means of most of the poor.

Cost of Medical Services

To test the assumption that the CSS participant group was, in fact, a random sample, we compared their medical costs for a six-month period to the medical costs of a random sample of California residents drawn from the Medi-Cal Paid Claims system. (Medi-Cal is the name of the California Medicaid program.) The average costs for the two samples were not significantly different, although the standard deviation of the random sample was higher, indicating that the CSS sample may have had somewhat fewer extremely ill members (Clark, Walter, and Miller 1982).

One way to look at medical costs is by the residency state of the individuals. Here, the two residency states are community—own home, board and care, in a relative's home, renting—and nonacute institutionalization in an intermediate care facility, extended care facility, or skilled nursing facility—all herein designated as nursing home. Acute care in a hospital is not considered a residency state, but rather a medical service used while the person is in either of the residency states. Community residents have medical costs while they are in the community—physicians' visits, prescription drugs, and so forth—and inpatient costs if they are hospitalized. Nursing home residents have the costs of residential care, medical services, and inpatient days if they have to be hospitalized. Table 6–7 data show the estimated monthly cost of medical services for CSS participants during 1981.

These costs are *estimated* costs derived from six months' data for each participant. Individuals could be in each group if they had both types of residency stays. For example, if an individual was in the community and had a hospital stay, he or she would be represented in the community-based group. If he or she then went to a nursing home, those costs would be averaged in the nursing home–based group. For a CSS participant who was in the community the entire time, the estimated average monthly cost for both Medicare and Medi-Cal services were $92.17 for nonacute services and $136.33 for acute care services. For nursing home residents the respective costs were $1,248.44 for nursing home nonacute care and $90.36 for acute care services.

The breakdown into service categories shows that for community residents, Medicare pays about 25 percent more for nonacute services. Medi-Cal's provision of prescription drugs is a significant proportion of its cost. A large proportion of the cost of acute care is paid by Medicare.

For nursing home care, of course, Medi-Cal is the primary provider. (In 1980, 50 percent of the total amount of public and private funding of nursing

Table 6–7
Average expected monthly paid claims, 1981, medical services

	Community Based		Nursing Home Based	
	Nonacute	Acute	Nonacute	Acute
Medi-Cal:				
Physician	$12.37	$ 3.94	$ 12.07	$ 1.88
Drugs	14.77	0.06	32.89	0.01
Other services	14.77	0.41	24.44	0.23
Institutional	0.00	22.40	1,083.40	29.71
Total per month	$41.91	$ 26.81	$1,152.80	$31.83
Medicare:				
Physician	$30.75	$ 8.30	$ 31.08	$ 6.31
Drugs	0.00	0.00	0.00	0.00
Other services	20.51	0.78	57.92	0.71
Institutional	0.00	100.44	6.64	51.51
Total per month	$51.26	$109.52	$ 95.64	$58.53
Total for medical services (not including out-of-pocket expenses)	$92.17	$136.33	$1,248.44	$90.36

Source: Clark, Walter, and Miller, "Estimates of Medical Services Cost: Medi-Cal and Medicare Paid Claims—1981"

Note: For CSS participants included in this dataset, the expected days per month in the community was 30.15; in nursing home was 30.17; in acute from community, 0.27; and in acute from nursing home, 0.25.

home care was provided by the Medicaid program [Gibson et al 1983]). In 1981, the average cost of nursing home care and ancillary medical services for CSS respondents was $1,152.80 per month. On average, Medicare provided another $95.64 in nonacute services.

Another way of looking at the cost of care is to show the actual costs during 1981 for the CSS participants by type of service. Data in table 6–8 show Medi-Cal and Medicare costs for acute care, community care, and nursing home care. Out-of-pocket expenses were not available from this data. However, the medical out-of-pocket expenses for all elderly in the western states was $130 (Kovar 1983).

The average length of stay for CSS participants in acute care hospitals was 10.3 days. There were 668 separate hospital stays. The average cost to the Medi-Cal program for each acute care stay was $762.45. This figure includes the deductible amounts for Medicare beneficiaries and the total hospital costs for any of the CSS participants who were not eligible for Medicare hospital insurance. The amount for drugs is underreported in that category, as most inpatient drug charges are included in the "institutional" category.

Table 6–8
Average total Medi-Cal and Medicare paid claims
for residency stays, 1981

	Medi-Cal Dollars	Medicare Dollars	Total Dollars
Acute Care:			
(Data consist of 668 separate hospital stays, with an average stay of 10.3 days)			
Physicians	149.28	330.80	480.08
Drugs	2.82	0.00	2.82
Institutional	591.56	3367.24	3958.80
Other	18.78	41.36	60.14
Total	762.45	3739.40	4501.85
Community Care:			
(Data consist of 1,825 separate community stays, with an average stay of 234.3 days)			
Physicians	75.76	168.24	244.00
Drugs	109.26	0.00	109.26
Institutional (Not applicable)			
Other	104.87	153.93	258.80
Total	289.89	322.17	612.06
Nursing Home Care:			
(Data consist of 130 separate nursing home stays, with an average stay of 140.6 days)			
Physicians	44.49	116.69	161.18
Drugs	144.02	0.00	144.02
Institutional	3789.22	341.52	4130.74
Other	580.93	296.62	877.55
Total	4558.67	754.98	5313.65

The Medicare program provided, on average, $3,739.40 for an acute stay. The total amount (Medicare and Medi-Cal expenditures) represents approximately $437 per day of acute care.

Most CSS participants were in the community for the entire year. The cost to Medi-Cal for an average community stay 234.3 days was $289.89 and to Medicare, $322.17. The total represents approximately $2.62 per day of medical costs for community residents. It includes physician visits, prescription drugs, physical therapy, outpatient and clinic visits, home health care, and any other services covered by either or both the programs.

When they were in a nursing home, CSS participants stayed, on average, four and a half months at a total cost of $5,313.65. Nearly 86 percent of the cost of this care was borne by Medi-Cal.

The Determinants of Average Daily Cost. During the time CSS participants were assessed and their medical costs monitored, attempts were made to discover the determinants of medical costs. What personal, environmental, or historical characteristics of people were associated with medical costs?

Various regression analyses were used to examine the determinants of both Medi-Cal and Medicare costs by residency state—community, acute care, and nursing home care.

For both Medi-Cal and Medicare, a higher proportion of time in acute care in the past six months was a predictor of higher costs for community residents in the current assessment period. And, for each program, the daily cost averaged over the previous six months correlated with current costs. That is, the higher past costs, the higher current costs. Most personal and environmental characteristics were not significant. People who were more independently performing the instrumental tasks of daily living were predicted to have lower medical costs. If a person reported his or her health as poor, Medi-Cal costs were predicted to be higher, but Medicare costs were lower. And those observed to show psychotic behavior had higher Medicare costs.

The paucity of significant personal characteristics is consistent with other research on medical care use (Mechanic 1979). Individual success with and attitude toward health care seem to be the more significant factors in use of such services.

Medi-Cal and Medicare reimbursement for hsopital care is fairly standard for the room, board, and general nursing care portion of the cost. (This data is from a period prior to the enactment of DRG-based [diagnosis-related groups] reimbursement schedules.) But costs do vary among patients. Intensive care requiring extra diagnostic tests or an operating room and anaesthesia, for example, raises the average daily rate. The significant variables are determinants of these differences.

The proportion of time in acute care in the previous six months was significant only in predicting lower Medicare acute care costs. Once again, for each program, the average daily costs in the previous six months were positively associated with higher costs in the current period.

For this particular group, elders with impaired vision had higher Medicare costs; having more informal support predicted somewhat lower Medicare acute care costs. The latter variable showed a curvilinear relationship. As the amount of informal support increased to higher levels (on a scale of zero to nineteen, indicating the number of personal and instrumental tasks with which a person received informal support) the effect on costs leveled out.

Black participants in this sample had somewhat higher Medicare hospital costs. The number of chronic conditions and age were both correlated negatively with costs. The more chronic conditions reported and the older the respondent, the lower the Medi-Cal costs, although Medicare costs were unaffected.

Nursing home care reimbursement per day, like acute care reimbursement, is unlikely to depend strongly on individual characteristics.

People living in counties with higher rates of available hospital beds had higher Medi-Cal costs (the primary payor of nursing home costs). Also, those with higher frailty indexes (Miller et al. 1984) were apt to have higher Medi-Cal costs. The higher the past daily Medi-Cal reimbursement, the lower the costs in the current period. The number of MSQ errors and age were negatively associated with Medicare costs.

In another study examining *total* Medi-Cal costs (community, acute care, and nursing home care) many of the same results were found, although at that time cost information for the previous six months was not available (Clark et al. 1982).

Lower levels of functioning in both personal and instrumental tasks were associated with higher Medi-Cal costs. Those with larger families had somewhat higher costs, as did those who lived alone. And, older persons tended to have somewhat lower costs.

Event Histories

One set of critical markers in the lives of the old and poor can be represented by residency change—that is, the movement between community, acute care, and nursing home residency states. The two instituitonal states are the ultimate expression of dependency. Even an acute care stay with a happy ending—reversal or cure of a threatening illness—reminds both young and old of how it feels to depend entirely on others for help, even with the most personal of tasks. However, the elderly have long since given up the illusion of immortality and an acute care stay can be keenly felt as a harbinger of coming debilitation.

More threatening to independence, but less likely to occur, is a nursing home stay. One survey of nursing home residency estimated that on any given day, 4.7 percent of the elderly population are in a nursing home. Age is an important determinant here: for those sixty-five to seventy-four, only 1 percent are in a nursing home; of those seventy-five to eighty-four the percentage rises to 7. Of the eighty-five plus population, more than 20 percent were in a nursing home at the time of the survey (U.S. Congress 1984).

Most reporting of institutionalization is driven by program reporting: number of discharges per one thousand recipients, for example, or expenditures per recipient and per enrollee of Medicare or Medicaid. While such distributions are useful to see the relative expenditures on types of service or to underscore large categories of expenditures, they rarely treat the interdependence of such residency stays or illuminate the individual case.

Of interest to the social and medical services are the determinants of such care. Is there a way to predict who will enter, and how often? One way is to look at the characteristics of those in one state or the other. When California was designing the Multipurpose Senior Services Project, experts sought to find the determinants of nursing home care, since the goal was to reduce nursing home days. In perusing the literature, they found many studies that focused on varying characteristics of nursing home residents upon entrance. Age, gender, recent illness, loss of a spouse, and so forth were all important variables in differentiating between those who did and did not enter nursing homes. However, when focusing on the Medicaid population, they found that 95 percent of recipients fit the profile of those most at risk of nursing home entrance. Because only 20 percent of the elderly population enters a nursing home at any time, these variables may describe "at risk," but do little to enlighten us as to who has the highest probability of actually entering a nursing home.

One way of studying change is through an event history analysis (Allison 1984). An event history is a longitudinal record of the exact time that certain events occurred. Rather than looking at a group of people at one particular time to discover whether the event occurred, we study a group of people over time, noting whether and when the event occurred. In the case of the CSS sample, events are changes from one residency state to another—community to hospital, nursing home to community, for example. We are interested in the number and type of events.

Also, an examination of an event history, combined with personal and environmental characteristics, permits exploration of possible causes of the events. The type of event history analysis in the examination of the CSS sample provides transition rates, here interpreted as the probability of going to a particular residency state in a given time period. While we do not examine the actual transition rates here, the analyses that produced the algorithm for determining rates permits us to examine the physical and environmental characteristics associated with different types of transitions. This analysis goes further than determining "at risk;" it examines the actual probability of transitions.

Figure 6–1 data show the residency states examined for CSS. There are three transitional states—community, acute care, and nursing home care—between which participants could move. There are two absorbing states—death and dropout. Absorbing states are those from which there is no exit, at least for the purposes of this analysis.

From national figures, we have the general approximation that about 30 percent of the elderly will enter a hospital during a given year, and about 5 percent will enter a nursing home. However, it is difficult to find a study that shows, for a random sample, the movement between all these states in a given time period. Given the fear that hospitalization and nursing home entrance are inevitable consequences of the aging process, we wish to see how often our sample of the old and poor actually made these transitions.

Figure 6–2 data portray some hypothetical event histories of elderly people. We are concerned here with only the transitional states. The figure

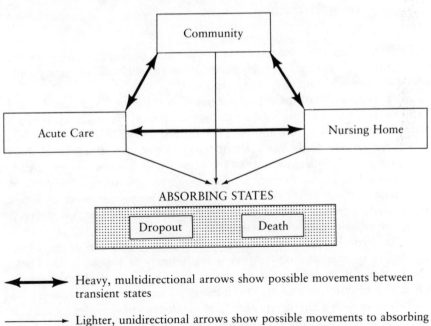

Heavy, multidirectional arrows show possible movements between transient states

Lighter, unidirectional arrows show possible movements to absorbing states

Figure 6–1. Residency states in the continuum of care

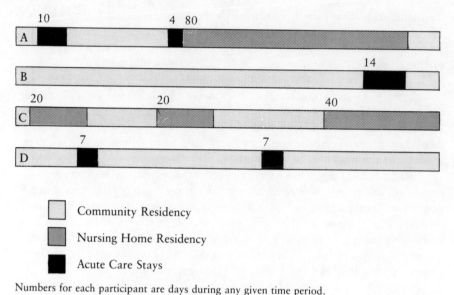

Numbers for each participant are days during any given time period.

Figure 6–2. Hypothetical event histories for CSS participants with residency changes

shows how summary measures of events—numbers of hospital days in a year, for example—obscure the possibly very different experiences of those people who have identical summary measures.

As a comparison of the event histories shows, persons A, B, and D have fourteen days each of hospital care in the time period, yet each represents a quite different set of circumstances. Each transition a person makes involves stress over and above the medical condition. A person with repeated short stays may actually suffer more than the person who has one longer stay.

Persons A and C have eighty days of nursing home care, yet their patterns also suggest very different event histories. While both seem to have, in this time period, a certain amount of residency instability, person A appears to be more medically critical than person C.

These hypothetical event histories are examples of our earlier suggestion that summary measures obscure what really happens for the aged. Those who have identical numbers of days in acute care or nursing home care are actually quite different and may need entirely different support systems.

Before pursuing the determinants of residency changes, let us look at some distributions of transitions. How much movement between residency states actually occurs for the old and poor? Because such changes sometimes have traumatic consequences, how often do they actually occur?

The number of people included in the distribution depicted in table 6–9

Table 6–9
Distribution of number of transitions, 1981–1982 (persons who were in the community on 1/1/81)

Number of transitions	Number	Percentage
None		
Remained in the community throughout the two-year period	561	45
Moved to an absorbing state (death or dropout)	122	10
One	35	3
Two	250	20
Three	27	2
Four	99	8
Five or more	156	12
Total	1,250	100

is somewhat less than the actual number of people in the sample. Some were not included in the event history analysis because incorrect identifying numbers precluded a complete Medicaid timeline. A comparison of those with complete data and those without showed no significant differences between the two.

As the data in table 6–9 show, in the two-year period, 1981 and 1982, of those persons who began the period in the community, 561 had **no** transitions. They may have moved in the community, but they did not have an institutional stay. Another 122 moved to an absorbing state—they died or dropped out of participation in the sample. Together, they represent 55 percent of the sample.

Three percent had one transition; that is, they moved into an institution and stayed. By far the largest number with any transitions had two transitions, typically going to the hospital and then returning to their homes. The next largest group had five or more transitions and represent persons with unstable or fairly critical conditions.

Table 6–10 presents the result of a regression analysis that investigated the effects of personal characteristics on transitions. The dependent variable is number of transitions. The statistically significant variables are shown in bold.

Race or ethnicity was significant, even with the inclusion of other variables. The indicators for Hispanic and Asian were statistically significant, and the indicator for black was very close to statistical significance, but only about half the magnitude of the other two. All were negative, indicating that, for this California sample, being nonwhite was associated with fewer residency state transitions.

A person who lived alone had six-tenths of a transition more than a person who lived with others. Not surprisingly, those with more chronic conditions and who rated their health as fair or poor had more transitions. Men had, on average, half a transition more than women.

Table 6–10
**Determinants of number of transitions 1981–1982 (persons who were
in the community on 1/1/81)**

Variable	Parameter Estimate	Standard Error	Probability That Estimate Is Significant
(Intercept)	3.7703	1.4060	0.0074
Age	0.0083	0.0120	0.4902
Spanish	−0.6923	0.2697	0.0104
Black	−0.3478	0.2147	0.1055
Asian	−0.7787	0.3061	0.0111
Married	0.0123	0.2346	0.9581
Alone	0.6369	0.2074	0.0022
Chronic conditions 1	0.2368	0.2088	0.2571
Chronic conditions 2	0.1954	0.0711	0.0061
Education level	0.0957	0.0943	0.3101
Self-rated health	0.4025	0.1265	0.0015
Hearing	−0.3812	0.2533	0.1326
Vision	−0.1705	0.2206	0.2205
Sex	0.5313	0.1851	0.0042
ADL independence	−0.1492	0.1273	0.2417
IADL independence	−0.3110	0.0626	0.0001
MSQ independence	−0.0603	0.0574	0.2935
Informal support strength	−0.0556	0.0337	0.0991

Note: Variables whose estimates are statistically significant at $p \leq .10$ are in bold.
$R^2 = 0.1175$

Independence in the Instrumental Activities of Daily Living was associated with fewer transitions and those with more informal support had fewer transitions. IADL independence is measured on a scale from zero to eight, eight being completely independent in these instrumental activities of daily living. A person who scored a low three on this scale had, on average, one less transition than someone who was completely dependent. Informal support was measured on a scale of zero to nineteen, nineteen being the highest level of support.

However, the number of transitions is only one dimension of residency change. While it might be an indicator of an unstable health problem or an environment without much help available, it is more interesting to know where people actually went when they changed their residency state. How many went to the hospital and returned home? How many of those going into a nursing home went for only a temporary stay? When they returned to the community, did they stay?

Table 6–11 shows the distribution of destination states for the 1,250 CSS participants who began the time period (1981–82) in the community. As shown in table 6–9, 561 stayed in the community. Of the ten who went to a nursing home and the 559 who went to a hospital, what was their next transition?

Table 6–11

Destination states of CSS community resident participants, first three transitions, 1981–1982 (persons in the community on 1/1/81)

Of the 1,250 community residents on 1/1/81:
  561 remained in the community
   10 went to a nursing home
  559 went to a hospital
   23 died without entering any other residency state
   97 dropped out without entering any other residency state

Transition	Community	Nursing Home	Hospital	Death	Dropout
Second					
From nursing home to	1	3	4	—	2
From hospital to	489	49	2	19	—
Third					
From community to	199	7	253	14	17
From nursing home to	12	6	7	10	3
From hospital to	1	3	—	—	—
Fourth					
From community to	3	2	8	—	—
From nursing home to	2	3	3	1	—
From hospital to	214	21	3	21	1

Note: 1) Boldface numbers are those who stayed in last state, i.e., on the third transition six people who moved to a nursing home stayed therefore the remainder of the two-year period. 2) Because some records were lost due to Medi-Cal number change or lost data, numbers do not add up exactly.

Of the ten who went to a nursing home, only one returned to the community on the second transition. Two dropped out of participation in the sample; four went to the hospital. Three of the ten remained in the nursing home during the two-year period.

Nineteen of the 559 who went to the hospital died there. Two remained in the hospital and 49 went into the nursing home. Eighty-seven percent of the acute care residents returned to the community and 41 percent remained in the community for the rest of the two-year period.

The remaining two transitions can be examined in the same manner. Of the 490 persons who returned to the community after one residency change (remember that this represents two transitions), 199 stayed in the community, 7 went to a nursing home, 253 went to the hospital, 14 died, and 17 dropped out of the sample. When the third transition was from a nursing home to another residency state, 13 entered an absorbing state (death or dropout) and 6 remained in the nursing home. Of the 4 who, at the second transition, went from a nursing home to the hospital, 3 returned to the nursing home and 1 went to the community.

While these distributional tables can help us see the movement between residency states, they do not help us understand the effects of personal and environmental characteristics on these movements. Are Judy Anderson or Agnes Hughes or any of the others we meet in this book in danger of institutionalization? Can we discriminate between groups better than just saying the older, white widow is the most likely to be in a nursing home?

This is the point at which event history becomes an important analytic tool. By using the methods described by Nancy Tuma and her associates (1979) and by Chiang (1980), the MSSP Evaluation Unit was able to determine the variables associated with various types of residency change.

Further, the mathematical properties of the method permits the estimation of the number of days in each residency state that can be expected in some time period for persons of differing personal characteristics. Since one of the major problems in social service programs is getting the services to the people who need them most, the results of these analyses could provide useful targeting information for programs whose goal is to reduce institutionalization.

Tables 6–12 through 6–14 show the general results of the analysis of residency changes. For our purposes here, we are interested in the variables that were statistically significant in the prediction of each type of change. The details of the method and the results may be found in Miller *et al.* (1984).

Table 6–12 data report the determinants of transition *from* the community to two residency states—hospital and nursing home—and one absorbing state—death. Our interest is in the variables associated with the transitions and their direction of effect. They either increase or inhibit the chances of transition. Another way to view it is to realize that increasing the transition rate means moving faster from the origin state to the designated destination. Therefore, variables with positive effects reduce the time in the origin state and variables with negative effects increase the time in the origin state.

Entrance into a nursing home from the community happens sooner if the person has had past inpatient care and higher costs. Higher past acute care costs, more time in the hospital, a recent nursing home stay, and higher medical costs in general all increase the likelihood of going to a nursing home sooner.

In addition, for this sample, higher levels of education and a higher score on the selection bias measure increased the rate of going to a nursing home. (The selection bias measure was a proxy measure for level of impairment and dependence.)

Not surprisingly, those persons whose IADL and MSQ scores were higher (indicating more independence) stayed in the community longer before going to a nursing home. More informal support and more formal support (represented by IHSS hours per day) were also positively associated. Scoring higher on the frailty index (a measure of the probability of death) indicated a longer stay in the community.

Going to the hospital is problematic to predict, because it is often a result

Table 6–12
Determinants of transition from community to other residency states or death

Transition	Positive increments in the transition rate	Negative increments in the transition rate
Community to nursing home	Past acute care costs	IADL independence
	Proportion of past six months in acute care	Sum of MSQ correct answers
		Informal support
	Discharge from nursing home in past three months.	Frailty index
		IHSS hours per day
	Level of education	
	Health costs per day	
	Selection bias measure	
Community to hospital	Past acute care costs	IADL independence
	Proportion of past six months in acute care	Hospital bed rates in county
	Self-rated health	Selection bias index
	Living alone	
	Stress index	
	Health cost per day	
	Frailty index	
Community to death	Self-rated health	ADL independence
	Informal support	
	Selection index	
	Frailty index	

of a sudden, critical event. However, a number of personal characteristics appeared as determinants of an increased rate of movement to the hospital. As in nursing home entrance, historical (past six months) data provided information. Higher past acute care costs, more time in the hospital, and medical costs were associated with acute care entrance. Those who rated their health as poor, those living alone, and those with stressful events in the past six months were more apt to go to the hospital more quickly. A higher probability of death (frailty index) also determined a higher chance of acute care.

Those who were frailer (selection bias index) and those living in counties with higher hospital bed rates were in the community longer. As in nursing home entrance, the more independent persons were likely to be in the community longer before entering a hospital.

Those who died in the community were more likely to have rated their health as poor. They also had more informal support, perhaps as a result of family and friends increasing their help in the face of a terminal illness. Higher values on the selection bias index and on the frailty index were also associated with death. The only variable associated with slower rates of death was ADL independence—the more a sample member was able to take care of his or her personal needs, the longer he or she lived.

Of particular interest to programs established to help people stay in the community are the variables that were associated with shortened nursing home stays. People who lived alone (in the community) returned more quickly to the community, as did those with higher levels of mental functioning (MSQ). Higher levels of medical costs per day were a determinant of moving from a nursing home to the community at a faster rate, just as they were associated with moving from the community to a nursing home. This no doubt reflects the higher level of medical problems in the persons in this sample who had such transitions (see table 6–13).

The selection index (higher frailty) was positively associated with the rate of returning to the community, as was the hospital bed rate in the county in

Table 6–13
Determinants of transition from nursing home to other residency states or death

Transition	Positive increments in the transition rate	Negative increments in the transition rate
Nursing home to community	Living alone	IADL independence
	Sum of MSQ correct answers	Frailty index
	Health costs per day	
	Selection index	
	Hospital bed rate in county	
	Support wanted	
	IHSS hours per day	
	Socialization services	
Nursing home to hospital	Education level	
	Judgment	
	Sum of MSQ correct answers	
	Selection bias index	
	Frailty index	
Nursing home to death	Chronic illness 1	Selection bias index
	IADL independence	Hospital bed rate in county
	Frailty index	

which the respondent resided. "Support wanted," a variable reporting the number of tasks with which the sample member said they would need help was also positively associated with higher chances of this transition. The more IHSS hours per day to which they were entitled shortened their nursing home stay, as did socialization services.

For those who made a transition from a nursing home to the hospital, the following variables were positively associated: education level, judgment, the sum of correct MSQ answers, the selection bias index, and the frailty index.

People with more chronic conditions, with more independence in IADL activities, and with higher frailty indexes died sooner in the nursing home. Those with a lower selection bias index and living in counties with higher hospital bed rates lived longer in the nursing home.

Many variables were associated with increasing or decreasing the rate of moving from the hospital to the community. Once again, history of medical care is reflected in past acute care costs as a determinant of the transition. Of interest in this case are the number of variables that show the support system—both informal and formal—awaiting the person upon return to home: informal support, a high score on a social network scale, services such as IHSS, meals, transportation, socialization, and public housing. This confirms the notion that hospital stays can be shortened by making sure that services are in place when the person returns home (see table 6–14).

The proportion of time spent in the past six months in acute care and a recent discharge from a nursing home both are negatively associated with leaving the hospital for the community. The more independent on ADL and the higher the hospital bed rate in the county, the longer was the hospital stay.

The only personal characteristics associated with the increasing the rate of transition from hospital to nursing home were education level and the level of support the sample respondent reporting needing. But the following variables were associated with a longer hospital stay when the person's destination was the nursing home: recent discharge from a nursing home, unimpaired judgment, IADL independence, higher levels of mental functioning (MSQ), the hospital bed rate in the county, the selection bias and frailty indexes, and the amount of informal support available.

The variables associated with a more rapid death in the hospital were age, gender (men), the selection bias and frailty indexes, and informal support.

One way to use the analyses whose results were reported in tables 6–12 through 6–14 is to designate those people most apt to enter institutional care. While hospital care is obviously motivated primarily by medical condition, the movement to nursing home is more likely to be a combination of medical and social reasons. As programs are established to help people maintain their

Table 6–14
Determinants of transition from hospital to other residency states or death

Transition	Positive increments in the transition rate	Negative increments in the transition rate
Hospital to community	Ailments	Proportion of past six months in acute care
	Chronic illness 2	Discharge from nursing home in past three months
	IADL independence	
	Walks independently	Self-rated health
	Selection bias index	ADL independence
	Frailty index	Hospital bed rate in county
	Lubben Social Network score	
	Informal support	
	IHSS hours per day	
	Meals (hours per day)	
	Transportation (hours per day)	
	Socialization (costs per day)	
	Public housing (costs per day)	
Hospital to nursing home	Education level	Discharge from nursing home in the past three months
	Support wanted	Judgment
		IADL independence
		Sum of MSQ correct answers
		Hospital bed rate in county
		Selection bias index
		Frailty index
		Informal support
Hospital to death	Age	
	Gender (1 = male)	
	Selection bias index	
	Frailty index	
	Informal support	

independence in the community, the fact of increasing numbers of the elderly will force the programs to screen their clients to focus their limited resources on those most likely to benefit from community-based support. Nursing home care is inevitable and appropriate for some people. However, others can be helped to remain at home. Using algorithms based on the analyses reported here (and in more detail in Miller *et al.* 1984) programs can determine groups of people most likely to move sooner into nursing home care in the absence of other supports.

We turn now to the special cases of the old and poor.

7
Ethnicity

Arethusa Fuller

Arethusa Fuller, seventy-two, seems slow, round, and soft. She wears a deep purple, floor-length gown trimmed in hot pink, and a bright pink hair net and slippers. The slowness of this black women is a deliberate pace; the roundness shapes the smooth edges of a real lady, and the only softness is in her heart.

Arethusa suffers with a serious heart condition that does not allow much walking, perhaps a block and a half at a time. She is easily upset and over-heated, and experiences "bad spells" when large veins swell and throb in her throat and her heart beats "very fast." She lives at the El Bethel Arms senior housing complex, which is actually a collection of multistory brown and white buildings placed in a square in the Fillmore district of San Francisco. Arethusa has lived alone in the tiny four-room apartment for about twelve years and observed the construction of one of the newer buildings in the complex. "Before they built that one outside my window I could see across the parking lot into downtown. Now I just see the plaza area below and the city through that narrow opening between the two buildings." She lives on the fifth floor in a brightly decorated, sunny apartment overlooking an urban park of sorts. Below, there are redwood tables, small shrubs and a barbecue area. Her walls are covered with pictures of her children and greeting cards. Two large pictures of Jesus Christ adorn her two largest living room walls. In her bedroom, a classic print of Christ with a bleeding heart hangs beside the bed. On a small table below it is an altar covered with religious statues and some flowers. A small white dove glows among the array. Mrs. Fuller is fervently religious. She is a member of the Third Baptist Church just up the street. Her faith is her strength and inspiration. She says her devotion has provided her with gifts of vision and healing.

Aside from the serious disabling limitations of her heart, Arethusa enjoys relatively fair health. She needs new glasses and has not had an adjusted prescription in years. For health care she goes to the clinic at Mt. Zion hospital . . . "and I never rush myself."

Arethusa was born in Mississippi. After marriage, she moved to Baton Rouge, then to New Orleans, and then west to Riverside, California.

In Riverside the stress of an unhappy marriage and insufferable heat pushed her to just walk away. A move to San Francisco, where she loves the cool weather and lack of racial prejudice, helped her begin a whole new life. Arethusa was the third of nine children and spent a rural childhood caring for little brothers and sisters. She attended school until the fifth grade and worked on and off as a domestic until her own health failed. Now Arethusa has a young black woman, a live-in friend of her daughter, come in and do the chores. The county's In-Home Supportive Services program, funded through the Social Services Block Grant under Title XX of the Social Security Act, pays for this household help, which includes grocery shopping, cleaning, and a little cooking. Mrs. Fuller was one of the earliest tenants in the El Bethel Arms and her apartment is immaculate. She still exclaims, "It's disgusting when you can't do like you used to!"

Arethusa's mother, Octavia, died when Arethusa was thirteen. She and a sister, Mary, were taken by a loving great-aunt to live in Baton Rouge. Arethusa also remembers a wonderful mother-in-law who cared for her own first child, Octavia, during the Depression. Arethusa remembers that the Depression was very rough. There wasn't enough food. The only work was domestic and Arethusa worked for nearly nothing. Octavia was only two or three months old then. Two other daughters were born to Arethusa. Today Mary Elizabeth lives in Riverside, and Roxanne lives across the street in San Francisco.

Arethusa dearly loves her daughters and grandchildren and recalls the trauma of moving away from the deep south to Riverside. Her beloved mother-in-law, Elvira, suddenly became deathly ill. Arethusa learned that Elvira felt brokenhearted at the thought of losing Octavia. Arethusa said the hardest decision of her life was choosing between the well-being of her mother-in-law and her first-born daughter. Arethusa left Octavia with Elvira and cried herself to sleep for a long, long time. Elvira never knew.

The misery of the Depression diminished during the years of World War II, when Arethusa worked for a "lovely white couple." "You know, there are two kinds of white people: the good kind and the rough kind. People are just prejudiced. I hit them with prayer. The Lord can take care of all your problems. You need to be right in the spirit of Almighty God. Living is important. Money is nice but not everything. People are greedy and ungrateful. If they put God in front, everything will be all right. Let Him lead them."

Arethusa has experienced the power of religion in the lives of her friends and family. She tells a story about one of her friends. "I once had a girl friend named Floretta who was married to an African man and had three children.

He was mean to her and her mother was concerned. One evening at dinner he threw a plate and badly cut her head behind the ear. Doctors at the emergency room tried to report the incident to the police but Floretta declined. About that time I had a vision that Floretta would meet and marry a wonderful man who would accept her children as his own. Well, the African man left and never came back and today Floretta is married to this wonderful man. You know, the Lord fixes you to help others. The Lord will supply your needs."

Another time Arethusa prayed for a child for her grandson's wife. Doctors had pronounced her granddaughter-in-law infertile after she had tried several years to have a baby. Arethusa says, "I got down on my knees and prayed for a child. Well, she's expecting now and I'll be a grandmother soon. Fuller can get a prayer through!"

People call Arethusa "Big Momma" softly and respectfully and phone her from all over the country to pray for them. "It's a joy to pray for others, to know that they have faith in you," says Arethusa.

Perhaps Arethusa's most powerful religious experience occurred when she found herself in the presence of God. "A black Jesus child sat on God's shoulder and I could put my hands around his little leg. I asked if I might lift and place him on the ground. But he was as heavy as the corner of this building. God placed him on the ground and he walked to sit by the saints on a long bench. The saint on the end kissed his head. Then I found myself walking down a round stairway and felt oil on my hands. I saw a stream two feet wide at the bottom of the stairs and I stepped across the Jordan river. Right then a great thought came that I could lay hands on the sick. You have to be all right inside for God to give you something like that. You know, people who don't know me say there is something great and special in me. I reply, "'It's God.' People say that I am different. I can't help it. He fixed me up to help."

During Mrs. Fuller's early years in San Francisco she lived in the housing projects for the poor. She had been low on food for a long time. She searched her coin purse and found less than two dollars. "I prayed for God to open the door so I might buy groceries. I walked out to the street and toward the market. I suddenly saw a tiny red purse sitting on top of a candy jar display in front of the candy store. I took it inside the store and returned it to a very troubled shopkeeper. As I walked out the door I truly felt the ground move under my feet. I heard a voice saying, 'That money was to be yours. That was yours, Arethusa.' You know, sometimes you can hurt yourself, because I went hungry."

A life-threatening incident occurred to Arethusa when her heart failed and she was rushed to Mt. Zion hospital. "You know the basement of Zion is the last drawer. When they take you there you're either going to die or live. I fought and prayed to live. Well, my doctor says I died and they revived me with that CPR. I lived. Dying wasn't painful or bad. It was soft and light and beautiful."

On her good days Mrs. Fuller takes a walk, a block at a time and resting after each. On other days she sits among her plants, a television, a radio with the dial set for religious programs, a religious record collection, and pictures created by her daughter Roxanne, an accomplished artist who works in several media. Her painting of a manger scene is rivaled only by a treasured large Bible for Mrs. Fuller's favor. The Bible is protectively wrapped in plastic.

Leafing through the pages of pictures in her Bible, Mrs. Fuller observes, "There are not any black people in the Bible pictures. I'm seventy-two years old and I know what prejudices are. I have always taught my nine grandchildren to treat everyone the same. No matter what race. I believe in good manners for children. Mine spoke when spoken to and behaved. You can't rush children into growing up."

Arethusa Fuller is enjoying peace of mind now, particularly without the burden of a husband. Men are relatively problematic in Arethusa's life. The tapestry of her years has been woven by women, women like her great-aunt, who rescued her after her mother's death; women like her former mother-in-law, Elvira, who labored and loved and provided continuity during the Depression; women like Roxanne who lives just across the street and has herself taken in a young married woman who lovingly cares for Mrs. Fuller.

Although her husband may have been problematic to Mrs. Fuller, companions were not. Until three years ago, she enjoyed the friendship of Mr. Jesse Patterson. He was like a father to her children. He called her his sweetheart and Arethusa thought him a saint. Even in the hospital, when he was failing, the nurses commented on his grace and dignity. He died soon afterward. Arethusa loved Jesse and carries a small photograph among the others of loved ones in her handbag. His picture reveals an elderly gentleman with a gentle smile and kind eyes, wearing a camel-colored vest and hat, leaning on a cane.

Arethusa says Jesse kept his own place and could cook and sew. She remembers at dinner they would each have something cooking in separate pots. She and Jesse would take turns stirring each other's pots as they both could not squeeze into her tiny kitchen at the same time. Arethusa and Jesse were together nineteen years and she still misses him terribly.

Even though Mrs. Fuller describes herself as "not an out-in-the-world person," she knows a lot of people in the building and can easily join friends in the dining room for several meals a week.

But for now, Arethusa is comfortable in her neatly scrubbed apartment. In a totally pink bathroom, neat stockpiles of hand soap and tissues occupy a space next to lines of freshly washed girdles drying on the tub. In the bedroom a raised bed is covered by a mat to protect sheets from body lotion.

Arethusa believes in cleanliness. She even scrubbed the stairs and landing of her flat in New Orleans because people sat on it all the time.

Mrs. Fuller looks into her open left hand like a book and, running her right index finger across an invisible line, says. "You know, the Lord has brought me a long ways. Even when I cannot get out I look out the window and watch for people who look unhappy or frowning. I pray for God to open the door for that person. They don't know it, yet I'm doing something even while just sitting here."

Rhea Majian

Rhea Majian may not have been able to make arrangements for her comfortable old age but her mother did. At age seventy-five, Rhea now lives in the family home in one of the better sections of San Francisco enjoying the accumulated family treasures reconstructed in America after a horrific past.

Rhea sits snugly on a brocade antique French love seat and gazes out a sunny window overlooking the lawn. She is perfectly groomed, with a short bouffant fresh from the hairdresser and a touch of bright lipstick and eye shadow. Her soft blouse and delicate crochet top provide a contrast to a heavy tweed skirt. Rhea holds her head and shoulders high and her eyes are resolute. Rhea Majian is a proud Armenian woman.

"I was a child of the Turkish genocide against the Armenians," are the first words she says to me. In May, 1915 when Rhea was four years old, she witnessed the massacre of her village in Armenia.

The Turks invaded the village and captured every man and boy over the age of adolescence. The men were bound and forced to stand in a line facing the women. The Turks then took a farming scythe and went along the line decapitating the men.

Mercifully, Rhea's father managed to escape. However, during flight from the village he was discovered by Turkish soldiers one evening. Mirhan Mirrijanian, the father of three daughters and one son, the wealthy merchant of Moush and Erzurum, simply disappeared, never to be seen or heard from again.

Rhea's life had not started out with such horror. She was born Heranoush Mirrijanian, the youngest of three sisters. Agnes is the middle sister. Ardemiss died several years ago. Rhea's family on both sides were among the wealthiest people in Moush, Armenia. Today, Moush has all but disappeared from the map. Only the village's geographic area—the Daron Valley—remains. Her father owned a slaughter house and specialized in fillet cured with garlic and spices. He sealed the meat in five-gallon containers and shipped goods all around Turkey. He was a leather merchant and also exported sugar.

Rhea's family resided in the village of Moush until her father made arrangements for them to join him with the business in another village in 1907. Rhea remembers a life filled with maids and nannies, one in which wealthy women did not have to toil.

In Armenia in those days a family's wealth was worn in gold and jewelry and rarely taken off, even in the public bath. Rhea laughed when she recalled that village people would inquire as to when members of her family planned to visit the communal bath, so they could attend too and look at all the wonderful jewelry. That jewelry helped save her family as her mother and sisters fled across the country from the Turks. It served as payment and bribes to buy safe passage through hostile towns and villages. Unfortunately the jewelry was almost useless for small purchases such as food, clothing, and other essentials. At the start of the escape, Turkish invaders only allowed one horse or donkey cart per family and all wordly goods had to fit into the cart, or be left behind. Rhea's mother and sister had one wagon and a half-dead horse. A servant helped care for the family and prepared a camp every night.

Many people suffered and died along the way. Shoes wore out and people wrapped their feet in rags. For food, families dug for wild or overlooked roots or leftover crops on the outskirts of villages. A frequent meal consisted of a stew made of watermelon and slaughtered animal blood. Because Rhea was a sturdy, courageous girl she was assigned by her mother the grisly task of locating animal slaughter sites and soaking up the blood and bits of remains with rags, to be later boiled in the stew. Rhea said the task turned her stomach, but the thought of her more delicate and hungry sisters gave her resolve.

The family's bribed its way across Turkey to get to Syria. All the children had money belts filled with gold coins for bribes. Unfortunately, the purchase of safe passage cost more than anticipated and Rhea's family ran out of money in Idina, Syria. Rhea's tiny family of women feared for their safety and lives.

Once again, Rhea's mother took charge. She placed the girls in a German orphanage and went to work as a charwoman in Aleppo, Syria. "My mother worked as a housekeeper and did washing for a year to earn passage to Istanbul." It took six months for Rhea's mother to save enough money to recover her children. Rhea said that during that time the women and the children were whipped and beaten by Turkish soldiers, but at least none of the women was raped. Rhea and her sisters were well treated in the orphanage.

At last the family arrived is Istanbul, where Rhea's mother was supposed to recover money and jewels from a bank, sent ahead for safekeeping by her father before his capture and death.

"Turkish bankers would not return all of our money and jewels. Only after a great deal of struggle and negotiation was my mother able to recover a little of the money. My father had also sent ahead valuable rugs to the

American Catholic missionaries in Istanbul for safekeeping. My mother also tried to recover our rugs as we were desperate. The missionaries were as uncooperative as the bankers. They said the rugs were lost and offered no explanation or assistance. I was nine years old then."

Once again, Rhea's resourceful mother searched for solutions and attempted to contact her aunt somewhere in the United States. An Armenian organization in America became involved and one sister was located in Fresno, California. Rhea's aunt promptly wired the family money and sponsored them to the United States.

Suddenly, on March 22, 1920, when Rhea was not quite eleven years old, the horror, brutality, hunger, and fear ended. Rhea and her mother and two sisters arrived by train in Fresno.

They had traveled from Istanbul to Greece, where they obtained passage to the United States on a Greek ship. Rhea's family was treated with respect and kindness by the Greeks, and they arrived without incident at Ellis Island in New York. Upon arrival Rhea had a spell of malaria and for a while it cast doubt on her entry to the United States. But it passed, and the family took the Santa Fe railroad to Fresno. Rhea has never had another malaria attack since immigrating.

"Mother was proud and took the last of the travel money and dressed us all in clean new clothes" Rhea recalls. "When we arrived at the train station a huge crowd met us. There must have been two hundred people in horses and buggies. We could not believe our eyes—we thought someone important was on the train. I think the whole Armenian community welcomed us to America that joyous day."

Rhea attended Emerson School in Fresno and there met an Armenian teacher, also named Rhea. Teacher Rhea insisted—even forced—the children to speak only English. She explained that adaptation and embracing American ways were the keys to survival. The student Rhea learned her lessons well. Sixty-five years later she speaks perfect English and is a loyal American, while at the same time preserving intelligent objectivity about politics. "I am terribly worried about Social Security and what will happen to the old. People have worked all of their lives and contributed and built this country, only to have no security in their old age."

Rhea was one of the immigrants who helped build America. She went to work in Rio Vista canning asparagus for Del Monte at age eleven. Family friends drove Rhea and her sisters to work camps in Rio Vista where they lived for two months while canning. When the season was over, the friends would return the girls home. "I'll never forget the day the inspectors came to the cannery. I could not speak English. The only way I could answer their questions about my age was to hold up my little fingers. The inspectors took me to the cannery office and found a translator. They told me I was too young to work right then and kindly suggested I go to school."

Rhea did return to a Catholic school in Fresno and received special treatment from the nuns. "The nuns took the children who could not speak English and separated them from the classes and taught them in a little group at the top of the stairs." Rhea went as far as the third grade.

Following her instruction from the nuns, Rhea again went to work canning figs at the Guggenheim packing house in Fresno. She was a skillful, hard worker and quickly became the fastest canner in the factory. She was also a graceful lady. She worked as a model for the posh City of Paris women's department store during 1926–1927.

About that time, Rhea's mother remarried and her new husband was a very wealthy man. The family moved to San Francisco. It was 1925 and Rhea was sixteen years old and earning sixteen dollars a week working at the Love Nest Candy Factory in San Franciso. They lived on Army Street, one of the better neighborhoods, but prosperity was short-lived when the Depression hit. Rhea's stepfather lost everything and the family moved to Northpoint Street, in the city's wharf district, where they lived for ten years. Rhea went back to work in the cannery at Fisherman's Wharf, now a boutique and restaurant-filled famous tourist attraction. "We canned dried fruits in winter and asparagus, tomatoes, apricots, cherries, peaches, and pears in the spring and summer."

Rhea's labor paid well, earning her $160 a week. It was at that time of renewed well-being that she met Robert Sullivan, who was everything Rhea was not—dashing, worldly, Irish, and Roman Catholic. Robert Sullivan captured Rhea's affections and they talked of marriage.

Their union was not to be. "My family would not allow us to marry. I could not. I had to live by the old ways where you did what you were told." There was a family-arranged match. Her husband-to-be was twenty-two years older and living in Fresno but part of the Armenian culture. He was financially secure. Stephen Majian had already reached his middle years and felt the first signs of age discrimination in his work place at Godchacks Department Store, when Rhea married him in Fresno in 1930. They continued living in Fresno for three years until Steve was forced to leave his position because of his age.

Rhea and Steve moved back to San Francisco and bought a grocery, deli, and liquor store at the corner of Geary and Divisadero, which she would help run for twenty-six years. Living in a cool and relatively loveless marriage, Rhea bore two sons. "Before I married I worked as a model for six months for the City of Paris and loved it. I wanted to start again but my husband was very old-fashioned. He would not allow me to work and be independent outside the family home and business."

Rhea made attempts to work outside the home at Livingston's Women's Store on Grant Avenue, but was obliged to return to the home. It was a bitter return home, because Rhea had invested a year's work to become a top salesperson. "I left my husband several times struggling to have a small piece of my own life. I suffered a lot. My mother threatened that she would die if I divorced and shamed the family name. My husband did not change. I did. I remained married for the children and the family name—but I learned to stop caring."

Finally, it was Rhea's son, now a pharmacist, who came to her rescue as a liberator. His brother had been killed in an automobile accident when he was only six, so in an age-old confrontation, the only son defended his mother from his father's demands.

However, the emotional and physical cost of Rhea's life had been high. At age fifty-one, she suffered a coronary that required a year of recovery. Rhea and her family were living on Twenty-fifth Avenue and Santiago at the time, and Rhea believes the steep climb uphill to home was the final blow to her troubled heart. "I also think that the stress of my marriage and forced isolation added to my illness."

Family and friends found a house on level ground. The sale, move, and remodeling are all a blur for Rhea. Her son's and sister's families, including nephews, did most of the heavy work and painting. The family room downstairs served as a makeshift kitchen while kitchen remodeling was completed. Rhea vividly remembers the now-covered original purple and plum wall paint and bouquets of lilies all over the house the day she moved in.

Rhea now lives alone and slowly cleans upstairs and then downstairs. Her sister, son, nephews, and friends fill the house daily but the use and traffic never show in Rhea's French Provençal showplace. Rhea invested and purchased wisely in the 1940s when her family income was prosperous and passed her good fortune along to her family. Today, with a meager income, she lives with treasures of the past.

Rhea buried her mother in 1946 after a lifetime of struggle, compounded by a second marriage late in life that did not work out. Rhea's younger and only living sister now lives nearby in Park Merced. A widow herself, she visits often and brews thick, black, sweet Armenian coffee. Rhea's son, Vahan, has helped her locate a physician to maintain otherwise good health. He joins her for lunch almost daily.

Rhea's husband died three years ago after a long illness requiring home nursing care. He left his entire estate to his sisters.

Today, Rhea is completely immersed in Armenian culture, society, and community service. She is a member of the Armenian American Citizens' League and gave the welcoming speech in May 1985. She works to support an Armenian Home for the Aged in Fresno, sponsors an athletic scholarship, contributes to an Armenian cultural society, and fosters an Armenian Relief society. She is a member of St. Gregory Apostolic Church, was president of the church board in 1952, and served for six years. In 1981 she served as president of the Ladies Auxiliary.

She looks forward to attending a special scholarship tea to raise money for education. "You know that I am very grateful to be in this country. Education is our pride. We did not have it and it is very valuable and important. We must not let educational programs and Social Security be cut by politicians. I like to be in public and love people. I even entertain a lot and love it too."

While explaining her love of community service, Rhea Majian's fingers are busy organizing a mailing for the scholarship tea.

Description and Analysis

These next sections look at what influence ethnicity may have on various dimensions of the lives of the ethnic minorities among the old and poor. Specifically, we look at three minority groups—blacks, Hispanics, and Asians—and compare them with whites along various dimensions. These dimensions include demographics, functional status, family structure and interaction, and use of informal support and formal services. In this chapter we try to provide an answer to the fundamental question posed by Vern Bengtson (1979): Does ethnicity make a difference in mitigating problems of growing old? In the context of our analysis, we paraphrase this question and ask: How strong is ethnicity in explaining and predicting basic behaviors among the low-income elderly?

Cross-Cultural Considerations

The story of Rhea, with its rich cultural details, vividly reminds us that ethnicity is not simply a question of color but that each racial, ethnic, and cultural ancestral heritage is proper study for ethnogerontological investigation (Gelfand and Kutzik 1979). With this in mind, definitional and conceptual issues become paramount. Currently, no widespread consensus exists as to what makes up a minority group (e.g., some group with similar cultural values or some culturally homogeneous group that has experienced discrimination and been denied access to social goods and services such as schooling), or even what makes up an ethnic grouping (e.g., is simple ancestry sufficient for membership or must there be some level of self-identification with that group; and, if the latter, how strong an identification before membership is attained and how is that strength measured?).

With these problems in mind, we formed the definitional problem around those groups commonly thought to have experienced some discrimination and been denied access to society's goods and services (e.g., schooling), thereby limiting their life chances and opportunities. In doing so, we implicitly confirm dominant group membership to the whites, which we know not to be true in all cases. Again Rhea's story speaks for itself: being white does not in and of itself guarantee anything.

While we group the CSS respondents in the four racial/ethnic subsamples of "white," "black," "Hispanic," and "Asian," we are aware that this approach has several limitations, particularly when exploring for differences between these particular groups. The major limitation is that such an aggregation is too gross and hides differences attributable to intra-racial or intra-ethnic factors. For example, how reasonable is it to expect that a white, Jewish, émigré widow behaves like Rhea Majian or like Judy Anderson from chapter 3, although all three are white, female, low-income widows? The question is equally applicable to the behaviors of a Hispanic born in Mexico and recently arrived to the United States when compared to a Hispanic born and raised in East Los Angeles and who has never left the area. Obviously, cultural differences exist and affect our results.

In the face of what might become irreducible pluralities of incommensurable behaviors and overwhelmed by relativistic analytic paralysis we chose to proceed with these four ethnic/racial groupings. Our expectation is that by ordering our observations in this manner some light can be shed on the conditions of these different ethnic groups. Whatever cross-cultural insensitivities we have committed, our decision was guided by Sir Francis Bacon's observation that truth is more likely to emerge from error than it is from confusion.

Base-line Demographic and Functional Data

As table 7–1 data show, the majority of blacks are in the San Francisco Bay area (San Francisco and Oakland), as are the Asians. Hispanics are mostly in the East Los Angeles area. The most culturally diverse area is San Francisco, while Santa Cruz and Eureka, our two smallest and least urban sites, are the most culturally homogeneous.

Table 7–2 presents baseline demographic and functional status data. Striking similarities of mean age between racial groups (no statistically significant differences at the $p. \leq .05$ level using a Chi square test) lends credence to the belief that elders of minority groups are a "biological elite." In fact, blacks seventy-five years old and older have lower mortality rates than whites. Whatever enables these elders to survive high infant-mortality rates of minority groups and pass through the rigors of childhood and adolescence seems to have guaranteed them a relatively "normal" life span. Jacquelyne Johnson Jackson (1982) points out that aged blacks tend to die, on average, earlier than aged whites (both sexes) but that the black male mortality rate is lower than for white males after age seventy-five. This crossover gap between white and black men over seventy-five years old widens over time.

Table 7–1
Distribution of ethnic/racial groups among CSS sampling sites

	Ethnic/Racial Groups[a]							
	White		*Black*		*Hispanic*		*Asian*[b]	
Site	M (235)	F (614)	M (71)	F (168)	M (32)	F (97)	M (37)	F (69)
Oakland	23	66	38	115	5	19	4	17
Santa Cruz	9	32	0	0	0	0	0	0
East Los Angeles	6	22	3	2	15	33	0	5
West Los Angeles	68	211	3	6	1	10	1	2
Long Beach	54	117	3	12	5	12	0	0
San Francisco	41	61	21	18	2	19	32	44
San Diego	22	66	2	5	4	4	0	1
Eureka	12	29	1	0	0	0	0	0

[a]Other groups, such as American Indian and Filipino, were excluded because of small cell size
[b]Chinese, Japanese, Korean

Living arrangement brings out one of the themes which we will see again in this chapter: whites and blacks tend to be more similar to each other, while Hispanics and Asians tend to be more similar. In this particular case, whites and blacks tend to live alone—as did Arethusa and Rhea—whereas the opposite is true for Hispanics and Asians.

Another case of striking similarities between whites and blacks, in contrast to Hispanics and Asians, deals with the marital status of men, seen in chapter 4, table 4–2. In this regard, white and black males are much less likely to be married than are the Hispanic and Asian males.

Educational levels also begin to bring out some of the differences in life choices that minority persons faced or that were made for them. The most pronounced difference is that while over half of the whites achieved an educational level of high school or beyond, over half of the Asians (Chinese and Japanese) had no formal schooling. What this may mean is that many of the ethnic minorities with little or no formal schooling may be functionally illiterate in two languages: English as well as their own first language.

The educational attainment levels may explain marked differences in the mental impairment status scores. The index used to calculate these levels is the Short Portable Mental Status Questionnaire, a ten-item list that measures intellectual impairment and is adjusted for educational level and race. Its developers created the racial adjustment based on samples of white and black elders in Durham County, North Carolina and we suspect the adjustment is not sufficiently sensitive for Asians or newly arrived immigrants. Our suspicions are based on reports from our Chinese and Japanese interviewers who felt that over three-quarters of their Asian respondents had an "intact" *functional* intellectual capability that is not reflected by this index. In other words, Asian respondents knew what they had to know. The SPMSQ may

Table 7–2
Percentage distributions of baseline demographic and functional data, by ethnic/racial groups

| | Ethnic/Racial Groups[a] | | | | | | | |
| | White | | Black | | Hispanic | | Asian[b] | |
	M (235)	F (614)	M (71)	F (168)	M (32)	F (97)	M (37)	F (69)
Age:				Percentage				
65–74	46.0	35.2	56.3	50.6	40.6	36.1	46.0	33.3
75–84	38.3	40.1	33.8	31.6	31.3	37.1	40.5	47.9
85+	15.7	24.7	9.9	17.8	28.1	26.8	13.5	18.8
				Years				
Average Age:	75.7	77.9	73.8	75.4	75.2	75.4	74.7	76.9
Standard Deviation:	7.0	8.0	5.6	7.1	6.4	7.1	5.3	7.2
Marital Status:				Percentage				
Married	42.0	13.0	33.0	11.0	72.0	17.0	76.0	29.0
Widowed	24.0	68.0	29.0	64.0	19.0	63.0	16.0	69.0
Sep./Div.	23.0	15.0	23.0	23.0	0.0	12.0	3.0	1.0
Single	11.0	4.0	15.0	2.0	9.0	8.0	5.0	1.0
Living Arrangement:				Percentage				
Alone	40.9	57.8	49.3	60.7	18.8	40.2	27.0	36.2
With others	59.1	42.2	50.7	29.3	81.2	59.8	73.0	63.8
Number of Children:				Percentage				
0	34	23	42	39	19	19	16	3
1	19	23	19	26	19	13	22	22
2	18	23	9	15	16	17	11	20
3	14	14	10	6	6	14	5	25
4+	16	17	20	14	59	37	47	30
Mean number	1.8	2.0	1.9	1.6	3.3	3.5	3.2	3.0
Number of Grandchildren:				Percentage				
0	23	15	39	29	7	9	14	3
1–4	40	41	22	28	26	19	26	29
5+	37	44	39	43	67	72	60	68
Mean number	6.0	6.4	9.3	9.0	10.1	14.2	7.8	9.2
Educational Level:				Percentage				
None	1.7	3.4	15.5	6.0	12.5	12.4	10.8	44.9
Grade school	35.3	36.0	56.4	55.4	50.0	54.6	40.6	43.5
High school	33.6	41.3	22.5	28.0	21.9	25.8	24.3	10.1
High school+	29.4	19.3	5.6	10.6	15.6	7.2	24.3	1.5
Average Years of Education:				Years				
	9.7	9.2	6.4	7.5	7.3	6.5	7.9	3.0
Standard Deviation	3.2	3.4	4.2	3.7	4.1	4.2	4.5	3.7
Mental Status:				Percentage				
Intact	81.7	81.1	90.1	85.1	90.6	81.4	86.5	60.9
Mild	13.2	11.4	8.5	10.1	6.3	13.4	8.1	23.2
Moderate	3.4	4.7	1.4	4.8	3.1	5.2	5.4	14.5
Severe	1.7	2.8	0.0	0.0	0.0	0.0	0.0	1.4

(continued)

Table 7–2 (continued)

	White		Black		Hispanic		Asian[b]	
	M (235)	F (614)	M (71)	F (168)	M (32)	F (97)	M (37)	F (69)
Number of ADL Dependencies:				Percentage				
0 (Independent)	89.6	77.6	78.9	74.1	84.4	81.4	81.1	88.5
1–2	6.4	14.7	15.5	20.5	15.6	11.3	13.5	8.7
3–4	3.1	4.4	2.8	4.2	0.0	5.2	5.4	1.4
5–6 (Dependent)	0.9	3.3	2.8	1.2	0.0	2.1	0.0	1.4
Number of IADL Dependencies: (for noninstitutionalized respondents only)				Percentage				
0 (Independent)	11.5	5.0	2.2	2.5	0.0	6.6	0.0	1.4
1–2	52.7	56.2	73.4	54.7	66.7	48.3	73.3	47.9
3–4	22.0	21.7	13.3	21.7	8.3	20.9	6.7	21.8
5–6	7.3	12.3	8.9	9.3	25.0	16.5	6.7	13.0
7–8 (Dependent)	6.5	4.8	2.2	11.8	0.0	7.7	13.3	15.9
Self-reported Health Status:				Percentage				
Good	41.6	38.9	36.6	39.9	43.8	33.0	27.0	39.1
Fair	44.2	45.4	46.5	42.8	46.8	47.4	56.8	55.1
Poor	14.2	15.7	16.9	17.3	9.4	19.6	16.2	5.8
Average Number of Chronic Conditions: (out of 25 possible conditions)				Number				
	2.4	2.9	2.4	2.8	2.3	2.6	1.8	1.4
Standard Deviation	1.9	2.0	1.7	1.8	1.7	1.9	1.6	1.3

[a]Other groups, such as American Indian and Filipino, were excluded because of small cell size
[b]Chinese, Japanese, Korean

be more sensitive at the more severe levels of impairment but it appears to be less useful, for some racial/ethnic groups, at the intact or mildly impaired levels.

The results of the SPMSQ highlight a measurement problem that occurs throughout this chapter to one degree or another and for any cross-cultural research:

> We may not be adequately sampling the cultural relevant skills. What we may be asking is the question, 'How well can *they* do *our* tricks?' whereas what we should be asking is, 'How well can *they* do *their* tricks?' (Dasen 1977)

Because our focus is on functional status, family structure and interaction, and use of services rather than on more abstract domains such as cognitive structures, we feel that although some items on the CSS questionnaire may be culturally "tricky," they do not confound the overall results. The probable exception may be the SPMSQ.

Our functional data show more similarities than differences (table 7–2). The Activities of Daily Living Index contains six personal care tasks such as bathing and eating and, as most elders are in general (Shanas 1979), the majority of all CSS respondents—irrespective of racial and ethnic grouping or gender—are independent in all these areas (here, as elsewhere in the book, "independent" means receiving no personal assistance in carrying out the task). The majority of respondents do need, however, some personal assistance in carrying out the eight tasks in the Instrumental Activities of Daily Living Index. The tasks needing assistance include shopping, travel, and meal preparation—the same pattern we saw in chapters 4 and 5. The overall level of dependency is in marked contrast to the elderly in general (Shanas 1977).

Both indices, ADL and IADL, are performance oriented (e.g., "Do you . . . ?") and the degrees to which independence or dependence in roles such as shopping are culturally determined is not known. For example, one respondent's daughter told the interviewer, "*No la dejo a mi mama salir sola, las calles son muy peligrosas.*" ("I don't let my mother go out alone, the streets are very dangerous.") To what degree this sentiment and similar feelings that tend to foster dependency—even if appropriate—is idiosyncratic to particular ethnic/racial groups is an empirical question that presently must go unanswered because of our measurement limitations.

From the analyses in chapter 5, we saw that ethnic/racial variables do influence functional status and how it may change over time. Being black was positively associated with decrements in the Activities of Daily Living (ADL) index while this was not the case for whites, Hispanics, or Asians (table 5–6). Also, being black was positively associated with lower scores in the initial Instrumental Activities of Daily Living measurement (table 5–8), as typified by Arethusa's difficulties with grocery shopping, cleaning, and cooking. Being black and Hispanic was associated with both higher initial scores in the Mental Status Questionnaire (MSQ) as well as with positive changes in the MSQ scores at the second interview. However, as we indicated in chapter 5 and in the beginning of this chapter, we are not completely confident in the MSQ to accurately measure initial impairment levels or changes over time, particularly for the minority groups.

What these results indicate is that some minorities do age at different rates then does the majority white population. (In this context, "age" is taken to mean the ability to carry out certain activities.) We see that blacks probably age the fastest, at least in terms of ADL and IADL scores, while Hispanics appear no different then the majority population.

In regard to health status and chronic conditions, we see all groups rate their health less well than does the general elderly population. For example, in 1981, only 30.1 percent of the U.S. population sixty-five years old and older reported their health status as fair or poor (AARP 1985). The low-income ethnic group's self-reported health status (table 7–2) as fair-poor ranged from 56 percent (Hispanic men) to 73 percent (Asian men).

Consistent with this finding concerns the number of chronic conditions. The general elderly population reports, on average, one condition, while the low-income ethnic group reports from a minimum of 1.4 (Asian women) to a maximum of 2.9 conditions (white women).

Family Structure and Interaction

White and black women tend to live alone. Hispanic and Asian women tend to live with others. We know from our other data, shown in chapter 4 (table 4–2), that most of these women are widows, so it is not the case that Hispanic and Asian women are living with their spouses.

To avoid lengthy repetitions we summarize the material from chapter 4 regarding ethnic/racial differences, and the family structure and family interaction:

- All groups tend to be part of multigenerational families, particularly Hispanics and Asians;
- Hispanic and Asian men are two to three times more likely to be married as are the white and black men;
- White and black men are twice as likely to live alone than are Hispanic and Asian men;
- Hispanics (men and women) and Asians (men and women) are more likely to have more children than whites and blacks (both sexes);
- Black men are most likely to have no children;
- All groups live close to their children and keep in frequent contact, particularly Hispanics;
- All groups live relatively far away from their siblings and infrequently keep in contact.

What we saw from the regression analyses in chapter 4 was that the predictors of frequency of contact and the number of informal supports provided were mainly associated with measures of need and the number of children available. Ethnic/racial variables were not significant except in the one case of "Asian" being negatively associated with receiving informal assistance. From all these analyses we conclude that not much substantive difference appears to exist between the relative strengths or weaknesses of the informal systems in terms of ethnic/racial groupings. While one group may be more active than another, it is most likely because of the number of children rather than a culturally derived learned behavior specific to an ethnic/racial group. Differences between groups appear marginal rather than essential.

Use of Formal Services: Nonmedical Services

The CSS questionnaire contained a separate subsection that listed thirty-seven individual services provided through publicly funded social and medical programs. The interviewers went through each service and asked if the respondent had received the service within the last month. Over half of all ethnic/racial groupings reported no services received within the last month. Black women reported the most received, with an average of 1.04 services, while Asian women reported the least, with an average 0.17 services. As we saw in table 6–7, black was the only significant ethnic variable when explaining the number of formal services received (see chapter 6 for more detail on the use of social services).

To more thoroughly examine the relationships between ethnic/racial groupings and use of formal services, we carried out two regression analyses on ethnic widows. We choose widows because they make up a group of particular interest to the service-providing community. The first equation had the number of formal services as the dependent variable and only the minority ethnic/racial groupings as independent variables. We found that, in contrast to the white women, black women received more services, while the Asian and Hispanic women received less than the white women (all were significant at the *p.* ≤ .10 level). Overall, this equation explained 3.9 percent of the variance.

The second equation had eleven independent variables and explained 18.8 percent of the variance. The results are shown in table 7–3 and reveal a more complex set of relationships. First we see that black women receive more services than white widows, while Asian women receive less than white women. No statistically significant difference exists between Hispanic and white women.

One possible explanation for Asian women receiving fewer services than white women is that agency personnel who authorize services have instituted some sort of administrative barrier to access by the Asian women. We do not

Table 7–3
Regression results with number of formal services received in last month as the dependent variable

Variable[a]	Estimate	t Value
Intercept	0.261	
Black	0.378	2.56
Asian	−0.242	−2.89
Number of ADL dependencies	0.187	3.16
Number of informal support areas provided		
R² = 0.18	−0.101	−4.66

[a]Other independent variables entered but not significant at the *p.* ≤ .10 level were: Hispanic, age group, siblings, grandchildren; and number of children.

believe this to be the case. As we showed in table 7–1, most of the Asian women, as well as the blacks, are from the San Francisco Bay Area. It is through the county departments of social services that the most frequently used service, In-Home Supportive Services, is provided and the county departments in the Bay Area have a large number of minorities on the staff who determine eligibility and award services. In addition, as we stated above, Asian women reported no unmet need and two of the significant variables in table 7–3 relate to need, indicating that the county-provided services system, at least in this instance, responds to need.

The other significant variable in table 7–3, the number of areas of support provided by the informal system, also indicates that the welfare system shies away from potential clients who have an active informal support system.

Discussion

The topic of minority elderly has its fair share of myths, or more formally, of contending hypotheses. Our results will support some of these hypotheses, but will test the validity of others. For example, in regard to living arrangements, we noted that white women *and* black women tend to live alone, while Hispanics and Asians tend to live with others. We found no significant age differentials among whites and nonwhites. We did find differences in educational attainment levels. We found little differences in functional levels in areas of personal care. Minorities were more dependent in areas of instrumental care, although white women had more chronic conditions than did nonwhites.

Regarding the question, "Do minorities age faster whan whites?" the answer seems to be yes, some do, specifically blacks. In the context of our definitions, this finding simply means that blacks tend to get more personal help to carry out their basic tasks of life then do other ethnic/racial groups. Getting more help means they score as more "dependent," meaning they "age" faster, or become functionally dependent earlier in life.

Our findings regarding the family point out a fact that is sometimes lost in debates about elderly whites and nonwhites: *all* have active informal support systems and that their children keep in frequent contact. These findings lead us to believe that discussions about differences between white and nonwhite elderly and the support that they receive are discussions about *marginal* differences. Support seems to be a function of need and the number of children to supply it than it is a function of culturally derived behaviors.

Another of our contributions to debates about the situation of elderly minorities is that black women seem to receive more formal services than whites, while Asian women receive less than whites. The fact that our sample was drawn from those low-income elderly *already* linked to the formal services system by virtue of being Medicaid enrollees and recipients of SSI/SSP precludes an interpretation of this finding based on questions of eligibility determination. We believe, rather, a reasonable interpretation of this finding is that these widows live in service environments that allow for the exercise of personal preferences and that are positively responsive to their needs to some degree.

Jeopardy Question

After our review of our data, both here and in chapters 4, 5, and 6, and a review of a major Medicare study discussed below, we have to conclude that ethnicity often is not a major explanatory variable. We believe that income, gender, and even the number of children are stronger explanatory variables and that ethnicity per se does not make much of a statistical difference except in some limited but important areas. Because all of our CSS respondents are low-income, we have examined two major studies to determine what effects income may have on some key variables such as health status, disability, morbidity, and mortality. Lewis Butler and Paul Newacheck (1981) analyzed Health Interview Survey data and concluded that older persons of low income are less healthy than other elderly, although, not controlling for income, nonwhites report more disabilities.

More recently, Alma McMillan and associates (1983) carried out an analysis of all Medicare enrollees in the U.S. and divided them into two major groups: those without "buy-in" and those with "buy-in." Those with buy-in are low-income individuals for whom the state pays the Medicare premium and are called the "crossover population" because their health insurance coverage crosses over Medicaid to Medicare. This group can be considered the poor and near poor. Those without the buy-in can be considered the nonpoor. In each case where race and income were controlled for, those with buy-in fared worse than those without buy-in. "Faring worse" means greater rates of hospital use, greater expenditures, higher levels of morbidity, and higher mortality rates. For example, in the dry but precise language of this report, "[T]he higher utilization rates for the buy-ins very likely reflect, in part, their excess mortality."

This "excess mortality" merits further detail because it graphically depicts the argument about the effects of income and race and the following is adapted from the McMillan study:

The magnitude of the simple ratios attest to the striking differences between the poor (with buy-in) and the nonpoor (without buy-in) concerning the summary statistic, percent dying, and reveal the importance of income as an explanatory variable. Although a measurable difference does exist within

Table 7–4
Percent of study enrollees dying, by buy-in status and race, U.S., 1978

Race	Total	Percent Dying		
		Without Buy-in	With Buy-in	Ratio: With to Without Buy-in
White	5.3	4.9	9.7	2.0
Other	5.5	4.7	7.3	1.6

Source: McMillan, A., *et al.* 1983. "A Study of the 'Crossover Population': Aged Persons Entitled to Both Medicare and Medicaid." *Health Care Financing Review.* 4: Table 13.

the buy-in group between the white and nonwhite groups (i.e., 9.7 versus 7.3), the greater differences exist between income groups.

While we consider income to be a stronger explanatory variable than ethnicity per se, we recognize that poverty rates are higher among the ethnic minority groups than among the whites. For example, in 1981, the poverty rate among aged white men was 8.5 percent, while it was 23.6 percent for Hispanic men and 32.2 percent among black men. The disparities among women follow the same pattern, with rural black elderly women being the most impoverished (68 percent) of any group of elderly. While recognizing the uneven income distribution, our point is that, analytically speaking, income appears to be a stronger predictor for major health-related behaviors than does ethnicity.

That gender is a greater explanatory variable than ethncity is commonly accepted and one has only to look at the income distribution between genders and the higher poverty rates among women to be reminded of this. Other significant differences are found in marital status and living arrangement.

A variable not so obvious and seldom mentioned in the ethnogerontological literature is number of living children. When analyzing familial interaction (e.g., level of support and frequency of contact), number of children appears to be more important than ethnicity per se when attempting to predict levels of support and frequency of contact. All groupings appear to have fairly strong family support systems and differences between ethnic groupings are marginal.

Other researchers, when studying familial interaction, have concluded that there exists support for the hypothesis that age exerts a lifelong influence on some aspects of ethnic variation with advancing age (Dowd and Bengtson 1978). In other words, advancing age acts as a leveler of racial inequalities that existed in mid-life. Because our quantitative data does not go back to mid-life, we cannot directly test this hypothesis. However, the major differences we have seen in familial interaction can be accounted for by identifying the number of living children. Oversimplifying our multivariate analysis, the number of children, rather than race/ethnicity per se, acts as a "leveler" or "divider," as the case may be.

An important area in which ethnicity does seem to play an important explanatory role is morbidity and specific causes of death. As mentioned earlier, nonwhites of all ages and income levels report more disabilities than whites. Our own data indicate a higher rate of functional dependencies among blacks than among other groups. When looking at national statistics for cause of death, we see dramatic differences between groups and genders (e.g., black infant-mortality rate is twice that of whites; blacks have a 30 percent higher mortality rate than whites because of heart disease; black and white men have almost twice the death rate caused by influenza and pneumonia than do black and white women; white men have over twice the death rate caused by bronchitis, emphysema, and asthma than do black men and ten times higher than black women). As one would expect, these differences also appear in use of acute care hospitals. For example, the poor and near-poor have twice the rate of acute care stays with diabetes mellitus as the major diagnosis than do the nonpoor (McMillan 1983, table 12) but these differences are mainly attributable to ethnic differences between white and blacks (Jackson 1982, table 2). Our own data, in table 6–13, showed being black a significant determinant of average daily cost of medical care while in the hospital. This high average daily cost may be a proxy for blacks' being more intensely sick while in the hospital.

Whether the causal factors for these patterns are biological or cultural in nature (e.g., dietary preferences) is a question beyond the scope of this chapter. Suffice to say that in some cases ethnicity can be a chief explanatory variable, particularly in epidemiological studies of morbidity and mortality. However, to truly understand its role, income and gender have to be controlled for in the analysis.

Ethnicity: Does It Make A Difference?

We began this chapter questioning the strength of ethnicity when attempting to explain and predict behaviors among the low-income elderly. When reviewing our statistical data we have to conclude that although ethnicity does have a measurable effect in some cases, other variables have stronger effects. Going beyond our own data, we find that income is perhaps the single strongest explanatory variable, probably followed by gender, which no doubt has a strong correlation with income. When we look at familial interaction, the number of children is more important than race/ethnicity. On the other hand, race/ethnicity is important when attempting to explain functional dependence, and we saw evidence that blacks do "age" faster than other groups. Also, ethnic minorities of color have higher morbidity and mortality rates in certain diseases than whites. Overall though, we conclude that only in special analyses, particularly epidemiological studies, does race/ethnicity make much of a difference in a quantitative sense.

However, our two vignettes present a different dimension. The stories of Arethusa and Rhea instruct us that if ethnicity does not make a statistical difference, it surely *matters* to the individual on the social level. For example, Rhea's ethnic background provides her with a support network, a sense of continuity, status, and role. Arethusa's ethnic background has also provided her with similar resources. The particular cultural idiosyncrasies vary. For example, Arethusa has found prayer to be a particularly powerful coping mechanism—not uncommon among black aged (Gibson 1986).

Although the details are different, these two stories show us that ethnicity as a variable functions so similarly that measurable differences in social and behavioral outcome indicators are difficult to detect statistically.

8
Widows

Introduction

Most American women will live out their lives as widows. Currently, over half of all women sixty-five or older are widows. Annually, about one hundred thousand women join the ranks of widows.

Despite these impressive numbers, only recently have social scientists systematically begun to study widowhood. Our knowledge base is just being constructed. We do know, however, that the "average" widow who has not remarried is sixty-five years old, has been widowed for six years, and can expect to live an additional nineteen years as a widow (U.S. Senate 1985). As such, this means the average woman will have a final career—widowhood—in addition to her previous careers, or roles, as wife, mother, and wage earner.

To date, most studies on widows have been cross-sectional and not longitudinal (i.e., following the career of widowhood over time). Our own CSS data is also cross-sectional, representing only a point-in-time snapshot of these low-income widows. However, our data present a unique portrait of widows toward the end of their lives. Since the average age of the CSS widow is seventy-eight, we can project, based on national patterns, that she had already been widowed for nineteen years—the average total duration of widowhood before death. Also, since the CSS widow at age seventy-eight can be expected to live to eighty-four years old, she will have experienced twenty-five years of widowhood. Most younger, married women probably do not expect to spend a quarter of a century in widowhood but this is a highly probable outcome for many. What one can expect during those years is of paramount importance to all.

The most prominent of the initial studies on widows was done by Helena Lopata in Chicago in the late sixties (Lopata 1973). Her survey of 301 widows examined what happened to the roles of wife, mother, sister, family member, friend, neighbor, worker, and community participant in widowhood. She concluded that what happens to these roles was a result not merely of changes introduced by the death of the husband and subsequent events, but also of voluntaristic decisions of the widow and others in her social circles. In other words, what happens to the woman as widow depends on her own voluntary actions and those of her family and friends around her.

Interestingly, Lopata found that, generally speaking, the life-styles of the black and white women were much more similar in widowhood than they had been in marriage, mainly because of changes in the economic situation of the white women. In this context, it is poverty, not age per se, which acts as the "great leveler" in later life.

In a later study, based on interviews with 1,169 Chicago area widows in 1974, Lopata (1979) concludes that more important than age, income, or children is the combination of education and urbanization that influences the life-style of a widow. Lopata points out the two major problems in widowhood: loss of income and emotional difficulties. The first problem is highlighted by the fact that widows have the highest poverty rate among adults. The second problem is related to the involuntary loss of the spouse, which necessitates a psychological process termed "grief work." This process, which can last up to two years, enables the widow to reconstruct the self as a partnerless person.

Lopata underscores the fact that the early stages of widowhood are very difficult because of the organization of social life based on a "couple-companionate" world. This initially sometimes leads to feelings as a "fifth wheel" and to loneliness. Over time, the feelings of loss and loneliness are eventually resolved.

Demographics

At average age seventy-eight, the CSS widows are about four years older than their counterparts in the U.S. general elderly population (U.S. Bureau of the Census 1983d). White widows had an average of 9.4 years of schooling; blacks an average of 7.5 years; and Hispanic and Asians fewer than five years. This means these two latter groups are deemed functionally illiterate—a consensus exists that a basic literacy standard consists of five years of schooling (Folger and Nam 1967). For the foreign-born widows, many probably used means other than formal schooling to achieve some level of literacy so there is not a 100 percent correspondence between illiteracy and no or little formal schooling. Nonetheless, we can assume that the foreign-born widows on average are functionally illiterate in their native language and in English.

While the white and black widows tend to live alone, the Hispanic and Asian widows tend, on average, to live with others. All groups of widows are part of families with three or more generations and all have two or more living children who live close by (within one hour) and who are in daily contact. Daughters are the primary source of assistance for the widows, as they are for nonpoor widows (Stone, Cafferata, and Sangl 1986).

Life Satisfaction

James Lubben (1985) examined the life satisfaction among the CSS widows. In his analysis, he reviewed a series of studies related to life satisfaction and morale among widows carried out since Lopata's last survey and concluded that:

> . . . . when the widowed (which includes both widows and widowers) are compared to the married, the married are less lonely, less depressed, happier, more positive, have higher morale, and are, generally, more satisfied with life. When widows are compared to married females, health appeared to be one of the key factors affecting morale. When an overall conclusion is drawn, income appears to be a key variable and the one that accounts for the majority of difference between groups.

What this statement says is that it is the difference in income levels and health status that account for much of the observed differences between the married and the widows. In short, widows would score as "happy" as the married if they enjoyed the same income levels and health. It appears that most of the more recent studies, some using sophisticated multivariate statistical techniques, do not ascribe as much importance to the "voluntaristic decisions" of widows but rather on factors largely beyond her control—income and health.

As we know, the CSS widows have less income than the general elderly and are in worse health. According to previous research, we would expect the CSS widows' life satisfaction scores to be less than those of the general elderly population. This is the case, but barely. Based on a national sample survey undertaken by Louis Harris and Associates (National Council on the Aging 1981), the national average score for the elderly is 24.7 and that of the CSS sample, both married and widows, is 24.0. Among the CSS women themselves, married women reported a higher median score (24.6) than did widows (23.9), but the difference was not statistically significant.

When Lubben and his associates examined the CSS data to discover major differences between the married and the widows, they found the widows tended to rate their own health status higher than the married. In addition, the married reported more ailments (5.3) than did the widows (4.2) and the difference was statistically significant. Lubben found significant differences in six ailments "often associated with anxiety and depression" and which were more apt to be reported by the married women: nervousness, stomach pains, exhaustion, fainting spells, headaches, and dizziness. Because spouses are the primary support for the other spouse, the married women appear to be suffering from the stress of caring for older and more frail husbands.

Another area of analysis was social interaction, as measured by how many people the CSS respondent "saw or heard from" on a monthly basis. The major differences were that the married women tended to see their off-spring more often. The widows had more frequent contact with friends.

When examining what contributes to life satisfaction, the multivariate analysis showed that health status and functional levels were most signifi-cant. Social interaction also contributed but to a lesser degree. The status of widowhood itself was not statistically significant.

In sum, widowhood per se does not seem to have affected the life satis-faction levels of the CSS widows. Whatever the traumatic experiences under-gone at the death of the spouse, the CSS widows seem to have successfully completed the necessary "grief work" and are as satisfied with their life as their married peers.

Functional Limitations

As we discussed in chapter 5, CSS respondents were asked about their abilit-ies to perform the six Activities of Daily Living tasks and the eight Indepen-dent Activities of Daily Living tasks. Although 71 percent of the widows reported being independent—not needing the personal help of others to per-form the task—in the ADL tasks, only 27 percent reported independence in the IADL tasks. These rates are in marked contrast to the elderly in general. Among the general noninstitutionalized elderly population, 88 percent report being independent in the ADL tasks and fully 87 percent report being inde-pendent in the IADL tasks (Feller 1983). As the analysis in chapter 5 showed, being married proved to be a statistically significant indicator as far as posi-tively affecting change in functioning level over time. Consequently, not only are the poor widows more impaired than the general elderly population, but they are also more at risk for rapid decrements in their functional levels among the poor population itself.

Service Use and Changes in Residency Settings

As shown in chapter 6, little differences exist between the married and un-marrieds, male or female, in the use of nonmedical services. Overall, 33.1 percent received at least one service (table 6–2), which is a higher use rate than the general elderly population. Robyn Stone (1986) estimates that 22 percent of the total elderly had used community services during the preceding year. For the general elderly, the most frequently used service was the senior center (15 percent), while only 1.4 percent used homemaker services. For the CSS respondents, the profile was 20 percent using a senior center but 49 percent using homemaker services. No doubt this service use pattern reflects the greater incidence of functional impairments among the CSS respondents and qualifying for means-tested services programs such as In-Home Support-ive Services.

The analysis in chapter 6 showed that being married had a slight positive effect associated with the number of formal services received. This may sug-gest that the spouse plays the role of advocate in obtaining services or that a couple, each partner with a set of functional limitations, may need additional services to support each other. On the other hand, living alone also predicted higher formal service use.

The pattern of medical services use is no less clear. The unmarrieds have higher average expenditure levels than the married group (table 6–11), but being married is a positive determinant associated with predicting higher daily costs of hospital care (table 6–13).

Marital status did not prove to be significant in any of the changes in residency settings or number of those changes as described in chapter 6 (table 6–12).

Summary

In a sense, this entire volume is about widows, because most aged poor are widows. The majority of the CSS participants are widows (53.3 percent), so all of our findings are heavily influenced by the behaviors of these women. This chapter briefly recapitulates and highlights some of the major findings about the CSS widows. The major differences are the most obvious: widows live alone and receive most informal assistance from their daughters rather than their spouses, as do their married peers. Social interaction is at a high rate, so the widows appear actively engaged with their friends and families although living alone.

Service use patterns and widowhood do not appear to be statistically significantly related.

As the vignettes and analyses revealed, these seventy-eight-year-old women are resilient survivors who live autonomously despite multiple medi-cal problems and functional limitations. They are as "happy" as their married peers. The biggest constraint in their lives seems to be a lack of cash. More money would allow them to improve the quality of their lives in their last years.

9
Nursing Homes and Families

John Mattus

John Mattus sits in a wheelchair, his right side paralyzed, and although alert, can only blink and mumble through a string of drool. It is difficult to see where his body begins and ends amid his two-hundred-pound frame and the folds of loosely tucked afghan.

But out of this rubble of a man is growing an artist. He is now a painter who struggles with his left hand to create abstract images of skinny men in virile stances jousting with one another. Men with tall round heads like hard hats. Men who may be in the building trades at a construction job site.

John's wheelchair sits in a room filled with lilting Mozart and cut egg crates that serve as paint containers. He concentrates on paper taped on the oil cloth covering a long table in front of him.

To John's left and right are wheelchairs with other people attempting to put something meaningful into what remains of their lives. John is part of an inspired arts project called Pleasure Endeavors at Laguna Honda Hospital.

Laguna Honda Hospital is the San Francisco city and county nursing home and one of the largest in the nation. Actually, Laguna Honda is a complex of narrow buildings all painted a sea shell coral pink and constructed in terraces on a hill in San Francisco. Laguna Honda suffers all the dramas of a historic landmark: magnificent large rooms with wood inlay and beautiful tiles and roaches and rats. Laguna Honda also enjoys a dedicated staff and heroic volunteers, but never enough funding.

Lena Jacobson, John's sister, recounted his story in an almost empty cafeteria while silent August fog wrapped the pink buildings in wet white gauze.

The Mattus family was Finnish and orginally came to the United States to mine in Montana. An explicit goal of their father was to get out of the killing job of mining. In a poorly timed move, the family resettled in Idaho to farm potatoes. Then the Depression hit. Father and Mother Mattus decided to send Father to California—to San Francisco—to find work in carpentry, an old family skill. The elder Mattus succeeded and sent for his wife, one daughter and two sons. Lena will never forget the day they arrived and Father took the family for a roller coaster ride over Dolores Street hills in their Model T Ford.

Life was not prosperous for the little family but needs were met and bills were paid.

Mother worked as an inspector for Best Foods mayonnaise. She died at age forty-two of cancer and Lena became the mother of the family. In time the family readjusted but it was hardest on Father. He never remarried.

Young John Mattus took up his father's carpentry trade, married, and began a family of two daughters in San Francisco.

Carpenty requires strength and an understanding of the big picture of construction work. Carpenters are often recognized as first among equals in the building trades. Carpenters are routinely advanced to positions of foremen and superintendents on construction jobs. Carpenters also enter the private sector and become subcontractors and general contractors themselves.

Such was the career of John Mattus. He started his own business with a partnership of his father and his wife as a bookkeeper. Business was sporadic and seasonal but they struggled along. John and his wife earned extra money by living in and managing apartment houses.

Looking back today, Lena Jacobson cannot remember clearly what started her brother John's drinking. He was a likeable, handsome man. He saw no wrong in anyone. She is equally puzzled about the drinking problem that developed with her sister-in-law, John's wife.

But drink they did, and a lot. Alcoholism began to affect the business, and fiscal disaster loomed. John and his wife attempted to care for their two daughters between jobs. They often were hospitalized because of alcoholism. But tragedy roared in from a completely unexpected direction.

One night John had been drinking heavily and was apprehended by the police. Lena explains that for some strange reason John put up a fight and was severely beaten by the police.

His daughter admitted him to San Francisco General Hospital where he was diagnosed as suffering major brain damage. He lost all memory and it was a long, painful, costly road to slight recovery. The beating occurred in 1980 and John was not old enough for Medicare. Lena says the expense to the city of San Francisco has been enormous.

In time John was mobile and even looked good, but was penniless. He was admitted to Laguna Honda with a very uncertain future. His future was determined for him when Laguna Honda experienced budget cuts and he was discharged to a wife who wanted him home but could not manage his care.

John Mattus returned to Laguna Honda by way of three other nursing homes. Lena Jacobson lived through the experience of all three and believes that Laguna Honda is the best.

In the Garland Nursing Home John was always at the bottom of the care list. Maybe being six feet tall, two hundred pounds and almost helpless was the problem. In any case he developed an infected foot. Even then his care continued poor.

Next he was moved to Daly City, a town contiguous to San Francisco. Finding a nursing home bed for a heavy-care patient on MediCal in San Francisco is about as likely as finding screen doors on submarines.

Again, his care was poor and police found him wandering around in the streets of Daly City. The nursing home owner had taken a trip to Reno and left the patients unattended.

John was once more removed and placed in a third nursing home near Daly City. The fifteen-bed facility consisted of a main building and a duplex. Lena believed he received tender attention there, but his heavy-care needs were soon beyond the staff's ability.

What happened next is speculation on the part of physicians and family, but apparently John's beating resulted in blood clots. Two dangerous clots in his lung and leg rested like time bombs within his body. One moved? John suffered a massive stroke—his right side became paralyzed and speech ceased. Also, at this time, his wife's health took a turn for the worse. She has cancer and other serious ailments and is living with their daughter.

John is now sixty-five years old and back in Laguna Honda, confined to a wheelchair with a shunt in his brain. A shunt is a tube that diverts and drains cerebrospinal fluid from the brain.

Lena says her brother has improved and gives much of the credit to "Pleasure Endeavors" arts program. He is now using his left hand and has sold two paintings. The family used the money to fix John's teeth. His morale is generally good. Depression sometimes settles in, but out-of-hospital trips on the "Freewheelers" bus offers needed diversion. John likes to eat everything and a high point of his week is a Tuesday afternoon guitar serenade in his ward by a patient that visits from Clarendon Hall across the grounds.

Even after all of John Mattus's misfortune, he still finds himself immersed within a loving family that strives to understand, accept, support, and love him.

Lena visits every Tuesday and brings and reads the Sunday newspaper funnies. "It helps him to talk. I also help him in and out of the Tuesday art class." Lena is herself a commercial artist in San Francisco. "I manage my own time. My day is my own. I care about my brother. It was very difficult for me at first, but he was so helpless it made me get stronger. Our other brother and his wife visit John every Wednesday and we do more if necessary. My husband cannot visit here because it is too hard on him emotionally."

Lena was very upset about recent criticism of Laguna Honda. She reports that "the staff is good and pleasant and the nurses are fine. Many patients are difficult here and far worse off than John."

Reflecting for a moment on the long-term fate of her brother, Lena says there is not enough to occupy one's mind. "People just sit and look into space. They have lost the will to go on." The key, she believes, is volunteers—volunteers to lend needed hands would help a great deal. People with lesser disabilities have given up. "I watched one volunteer work daily for three years to pull an old man out of a death-wish depression and back into the world of the living. Today he is involved and smiles and has made a kind of peaceful adjustment. On the other hand, there should be a humane way out for elders where possibilities are too few and pain is great. That is torture."

But what about the here and now for people like John, for whom possibilities are growing, pain is diminishing, and family love is great?

Lena gazes over the silent fog and in a quiet voice of tender compassion explains that she and John's daughter used to do all the laundry and errands. That is not necessary now. She entertains him with slide shows. She is a docent at a museum and once guided a tour of the Freewheelers. Lena is very careful not to let her talent as an artist interfere with John's developing interest and skill. "I offer encouragement and companionship. I will be here for whatever he needs in the future. What we really need are volunteers to wheel patients into the elevators so they may come for studio time like John."

Introduction to Analysis

Nursing home care is an important area of study for several reasons. First, federal, state, and private spending for nursing care adds up to more than $30 billion per year. Total annual expenditures from private sources is over $15 billion. Medicaid spends more than $14 billion yearly. Medicare spends approximately $650 million. Second, on any given day, 1.5 million patients occupy beds in the nation's fifteen thousand nursing homes (United States Congress 1986b). About 5 percent of the population sixty-five and older, 10 percent of the population seventy-five and older, and 22 percent of the population eight-five and older are residents of nursing homes on any given day. Over a lifetime, it is estimated that about 25 percent of us will have at least one episode in a nursing home (Kastenbaum and Candy 1973; Palmore 1976; Wershow 1976). The combination of large amounts of money and the scandal-ridden history of nursing home care has generated an intense interest in the topic and volumes of studies and government reports are available. Vladeck (1980), Johnson and Grant (1985), and Vogel and Palmer (1985) have published the more recent and significant works on nursing homes.

This chapter focuses on a myth in gerontology that seems to persist in the "common wisdom" about families' care of their aged members and the use of nursing homes. The myth, in spite of findings to the contrary (Dobrof and Litwak 1977; Vladeck 1980), is that the aged are systematically dumped and abandoned in nursing homes by their children. Specifically, this chapter presents quantitative descriptions of the kinds of support provided by the informal support systems (unpaid family and friends) to skilled nursing facility (SNF) patients, and contrasts that assistance to support provided by the formal system (publicly funded social and medical systems). We also describe the family structure of the inpatients and the frequency of contact with their children. We found that the actions taken by Lena, her brother, and her sister-in-law are more typical than atypical.

Methods

Data are from a SNF admissions cohort identified in a period between 1981 and 1982 as a subsample for the California Senior Survey. This subsample is distinct from the noninstitutionalized subsample we have discussed in the preceding chapters. The nursing home respondents reported about were randomly chosen from Treatment Authorization Request (TAR) forms filed in regional Medicaid Field offices. Medicaid uses these TAR forms to approve payment and SNFs must have written TARs for their Medicaid patients to be reimbursed. CSS interviewers were instructed to limit their selection of potential respondents to those who were Medicaid recipients, were sixty-five and older, and were located within prespecified geographical areas.

As persons already enrolled in the Medicaid program, all respondents are low-income individuals by definition. In addition, research assistants were to select only those TARs marked "initial," as against those marked "reauthorization" or "transfer." An "initial" TAR meant the Medicaid recipient had at least a twenty-four-hour break in nursing home service. "Reauthorization" meant the person was already an inpatient and the request was for continued Medicaid reimbursement. "Transfer" meant the Medicaid person was to be transferred from one nursing home to another.

Therefore, our sample is an admissions cohort but is *not* necessarily a sample of first-time users of nursing home care. Although such a group would be valuable for research purposes, "true initials" (i.e., first-time users) cannot be identified from the TAR forms as they currently exist. Data presented here are from the first interview only. The mean length of time between admission and the interview for the group reported here was 63.5 days (SD = 36.6).

Results

Baseline Data

This section presents findings on baseline demographic and functional data. The data in table 9–1 suggest the CSS SNF subsample has a varied ethnic

Table 9–1

Percentage distribution of the CSS nursing home sample, by demographic and functional characteristics

Characteristic	Total 100%	CSS Respondents (n=132) Percentage Distributions Male 27%	Female 73%
Age			
65–74	18	17	18
75–84	43	47	42
85 +	39	36	40
Mean age at admission		81.6	82.8
Race			
White	64	64	65
Black	14	11	16
Asian	11	17	9
Hispanic	8	6	9
Other	3	2	1
Marital status			
Married	14	31	7
Widowed	69	44	78
Divorced/Separated	8	11	7
Never married	9	14	8
Intellectual functioning			
Intact	29	38	26
Mild impairment	21	25	19
Moderate impairment	28	28	27
Severe impairment	22	9	28
Walks independently	65	58	68
ADL levels[a]			
Most independent	14	17	13
Most dependent	8	8	8
Average number of chronic conditions		5.4	4.7

[a]"ADL Levels" is from the Activities of Daily Living Index (Katz et al., 1963 and 1970), which is a six-item scale that rates actual functioning levels in eating, toileting, transfer, dressing, bathing, and continence.

mix—36 percent of the respondents represent ethnic minorities—and that the CSS respondents are quite old. Eighty-three percent of the men and 82 percent of the women are seventy-five years old and older. By far, most of our respondents are widowed, nearly 70 percent. If we add together just women who are widowed, divorced, separated, or never married, the spouseless total 93 perdent. Exactly half of the respondents suffer moderately to severely impaired intellectual functioning. Average number of chronic conditions are 5.4 for males and 4.7 for females. In all, the CSS sample is very similar to the "typical" nursing home patient: an aged spouseless Caucasian woman with impaired intellectual and functioning abilities (United States Department of Health, Education, and Welfare 1981).

Family Structure and Contact by Children

Table 9–2 presents data on the family structure of CSS nursing home patients and reveals that most are members of multigenerational families. In addition, of those who have living children (71 percent), most of their children live within one hour of the respondent. The mean number of children living nearby is 2.6.

Table 9–3 presents CSS data on the frequency of contact of the children with their parents. This relatively high level of contact—78 percent had contact at least weekly—may be surprising to those unfamiliar with nursing home environments, given popular conceptions about "abandonment." Lena's pattern of visiting her brother John reflects this "normal" pattern.

We used regression analyses to better understand the frequency of contact by children. Because of the relatively large number of minorities in our sample, we first explored what difference race or ethnicity would make. We hypothesized that the minorities might have larger extended families, which could influence visiting patterns. Using only minority racial/ethnic groupings as independent variables (i.e., black, Asian, and Hispanic) we found that

Table 9–2
CSS nursing home sample respondents' family structures

	CSS Respondents $(n=132)$ Percentage Distributions		
Characteristic	Total %	Male %	Female %
Number of generations			
0 (kinless)	5	15	1
1	10	5	12
2	7	5	8
3 or more	78	75	79
Living spouse			
Yes	14	25	9
No	86	75	91
Living sibling			
Yes	48	47	48
No	52	53	52
Living children			
Yes	76	70	78
No	24	30	22
Average number of living children		2.6	2.5
Living grandchildren			
Yes	78	75	21
No	22	25	21
Number of children within an hour			
0	27	33	24
1	3	6	2
3	35	33	36
4+	7	6	8

Table 9–3
Frequency of contact[a] for CSS nursing home respondents

Frequency	Percentage Distribution (n=132) %
Daily/Weekly	78
Monthly	8
More than monthly[b]	14
Total	100

[a]A "contact" could be a visit, phone call, or letter.
[b]If a CSS respondent answered "none," then it was coded as "more than a month."

they were not significant at either the $p. \leq .05$ or $p. \leq .10$ levels. Consequently, we reject our hypothesis that minorities are visited more frequently than whites in our sample. We then carried out a regression on frequency of contact by children that contained twelve independent variables. Overall, this regression explained 37.9 percent of the variance and the only variables significant at either the $p. \leq .05$ or $p. \leq .10$ levels were age (positively; or, the older the CSS respondent, the more visits by childen); siblings (negatively; or, the greater number of siblings, the fewer visits by children, which seems to be the case with John and his brother and sister); and, grandchildren (negatively; or, the greater number of grandchildren, the fewer visits by children). The actual results are shown in table 9–4.

Table 9–4
Regression results of predictors of frequency of contact by children

Variables	Unstandardized Regression Coefficients	Standard Errors
Age group	0.581*	0.148
Siblings	−0.608*	0.199
Grandchildren	−0.419	0.367

$R^2 = 0.379$
*$p. \leq .01$

Other variables included but not significant at the $p. \leq .05$ or $p. \leq .10$ levels were sex; race; disorientation (yes/no); number of chronic conditions (0–37); number of ADL dependencies (0–6); and number of children within one hour.

Informal and Formal Support

Table 9–5 displays a quantitative description of the kinds of support provided by the informal support system to nursing home patients. This is in contrast to support provided by the formal system. When questioned about these areas, respondents or proxies were asked to choose from among the following response categories:

- does not need support
- needs support and is provided by the formal system
- needs support and is provided by the informal system
- needs support but does not have it
- not applicable

When faced with circumstances in which a respondent received both informal and formal support, the CSS interviewers were instructed to probe and code the **primary** source of support—no combination responses were allowed.

Table 9–5
Ranking of support activities according to informal support proportion for those CSS respondents reporting a need filled *primarily* by either the informal system or the formal system (no combination permitted)

Activity and Rank	Title 22 Mandated Yes/No	Number Receiving Assistance	Source: Informal	Formal
			Percentage	
1. Money Mgt.	No	92	66	34
2. Social network[a]	No	79	53	47
3. Travel	No	68	38	62
4. Laundry	Yes/No[b]	127	19	81
5. Outside mobility	No	60	17	83
6. Accompanying[a]	No	86	14	86
7. Telephoning	No	51	10	90
8. Stair climbing	No	48	6	94
9. Wheelchair use	Yes	53	4	96
10. Eating/Feeding	Yes	35	3	97
11. Bathing	Yes	102	2	98
Toileting	Yes	66	2	98
Transfer	Yes	66	2	98
Walking	Yes	53	2	98
12. Dressing	Yes	74	1	99
13. Meal preparation	Yes	126	1	99

[a]The difference between "Social network" and "Accompanying" is that the former is limited to visiting for social purposes and the latter is limited to visiting public agencies.

[b]Title 22 mandates that bedclothing and dressing gowns be laundered by the nursing home; laundry of personal clothing is the patient's responsibility although some nursing homes will launder the patient's clothes for a small additional fee. Because of this fee, many patients remain in their dressing gowns.

Table 9–6
Results of regression analysis of predictors of informal support

Variable	Unstandardized Regression Coefficients	Standard Errors
Spouse present	0.818**	0.478
Number of children	0.223*	0.109
Orientation	0.888*	0.405

$R^2 = 0.201$

*p. ≤ .05

**p. ≤ .10

Other variables included but not significant at the p. ≤ .10 were: sex; age group (65–74, 75–84, and 85 +); siblings (number of); number of ADL dependencies (0–6); number of chronic conditions (0–37); and grandchildren (yes/no).

We found that larger proportions of informal support cluster around socializing activities (e.g., social network and travel and activities such as Lena's reading the Sunday funnies to her brother) and smaller portions supplement the support for which the nursing home is primarily and legally responsible such as personal care activities like eating and bathing. Since respondents had a forced choice between the primacy of informal or formal sources of support, we were surprised that the informal support shows up at all in these latter legally mandated categories, shown as a "Yes" in the column "Title 22 Mandated" in table 9–5 (Title 22 is part of the California Administrative Code).

In regard to the question, "Who receives informal support?" we again began exploring for the possible effects of race alone. In a regression using minority racial/ethnic groupings as the only independent variables, we did not find them significant at the *p*. ≤ .10 level. We then constructed a model with twelve independent variables that explained 20.1 percent of the variance (table 9–6). The significant independent variables were: being mentally oriented (positively); having a spouse (positively); and, the number of children (positively).

Limitations

There are several limitations to our results that merit attention. First, we should keep in mind that ours is an admissions cohort and patterns described here may change over time for those patients with extended lengths of time. Second, our analyses cannot consider individual facility characteristics that may affect patterns of contact and caring. For example, does it make a difference if the nursing home is proprietary or nonprofit? Does facility size affect these patterns? Our data base does not contain these items and, unfortunately, we must leave these questions unanswered. Third, the small numbers in our sample who do need assistance and receive that assistance primarily from the informal support system prevent generalizations. On the other hand, our results are highly suggestive that families and friends are doing more underneath the roof of the nursing home than has been generally accepted.

Discussion

Our findings reveal patterns of continuing contact and support by the informal system. Because our interviews took place approximately two months after admission, special family behaviors that may be associated with an admission trauma should not confound our results. Informal support and family contact does not stop at the doors of nursing homes.

Our data reveal (table 9–3) that typical nursing home residents, contrary to popular myth, are **not** abandoned in nursing homes. This pattern of continued contact, visits, and work is further confirmed by a recent California Department of Health Services Survey of Medicaid nursing home inpatients, which found that 77 percent of the inpatients had family visits at least weekly (California 1983). Our overall impression is that the informal support system is active and works in areas beyond the responsibility of the nursing home and in areas that are clearly the legal responsibility of the nursing home.

Regression analyses indicate that contacts by children increase with the advancing age of the patients and decrease if patients have grandchildren or siblings. This suggests to us that as the child has more discretionary time and fewer care concerns (e.g., own children) frequency of contact will increase. Contact appears to be easier for the older child than for the younger child. In other words, a sixty-five-year-old daughter, whose husband may be retired and whose children no longer live at home, may have more free time than a fifty-year-old daughter who still works.

Presence of siblings and grandchildren, which negatively correlates with children's contacts, suggests there may be a division of labor among the family as to who keeps in contact with the patient. Perhaps as attrition affects the older cohort, the younger cohort continues contact. The statistical significance of the number of children and presence of spouse regarding the provision of informal support further belies the myth of abandonment. On the other hand, mental orientation proved to be statistically significant, indicating that there may be a certain "distancing" by the family that occurs when the patient is mentally disoriented and no longer recognizes the visiting family member. However, Lena and her relatives show no sign of distancing themselves from John and will probably continue their visiting patterns until he dies.

Overall, we did not detect signs that children are "dumping" or abandoning poor aged parents in nursing homes. Indeed, patterns of nearby children (table 9–2) suggest that children may influence placement decisions so they can easily visit. We have reported elsewhere about families' active participation in those placement decisions (Pelham and Clark 1982).

To be sure, one can "abandon" an elder and still visit and provide informal support. Yet such patterns are neither likely to be sustained over time nor likely to be the norm.

Why the popular myth of abandonment has persisted so long is intriguing. National data on frequency of visits have been available since the first National Nursing Home Survey, 1973–74 published its findings in 1977. These data indicate that 61 percent had visitors at least weekly (United States Department of Health, Education, and Welfare 1977). This phenomenon of contact and caring probably has been occurring since the advent of widespread public financing of nursing home care in the mid-sixties.

Our own speculation about its persistence is that perhaps all parties involved—patient, family, nursing home industry, and public funding agencies—derive some benefit from the myth. For example, the patient may find it convenient to invoke the myth to instill guilt in the child and assure continued contact; the child may find the myth a negative motivating factor for "heroic" behavior and to avoid the social stigma of abandoning the parent; the nursing home industry may find it a convenient continued justification of its existence; and public funding agencies may use it as a rationale for why alternative modes of care are not examined and funded.

Whatever the reasons, future policy debates about nursing homes should take into serious consideration the actual behavior of the family and not be guided by convenient but fictive beliefs.

A somewhat different version of this chapter was published by the Elvirita Lewis Foundation as "Informal Support Provided to a Recent Admissions Cohort of Medicaid Skilled Nursing Facility Patients," an Occasional Paper of The Elder Press, No. 407, 1984. The material has been used with the permission of the Elvirita Lewis Foundation. The Elder Press is the publishing division of the Elvirita Lewis Foundation, Suite 144, Airport Park Plaza, 255 N. El Cielo Road, Palm Springs, Calif., 92262.

10
The Very Aged

Albert Shaw

Albert Shaw spends the greater part of every afternoon and early evening in exactly the same spot. He sits in a straight-backed wooden chair, on a soiled wooden hall floor, gazing out a dirty glass window in a wooden door, in a small, dirty, wooden duplex house in the flatlands of Oakland.

Albert Shaw is ninety-three years old, tall, nearly blind, cautious, black, and quite poor. He sits with his aluminum walker between his long legs and aching knees. Wrapped around the top bar of the walker is a once white—but now grimy gray—rag used to wipe glasses, nose, hands, spills, and then carefully rewound with two loops and a tie on the walker.

Venturing outside is possible with the walker but Albert needs an escort, ride, or taxi for transportation.

Born in Nacogdoches County, Texas, Albert Shaw lived 148 miles from Dallas and 148 miles from Houston—half-way between the two cities. Albert grew up on the family farm of two hundred acres with ten brothers and four sisters. His father grew cotton, corn, sugar cane, peas, peanuts, and potatoes. Albert was the seventh child of the fourteen. Six brothers and one sister survive. Two of the brothers live in Oakland and Albert sees them often. He proudly recalls that, "My mother and father *raised* us; there are seven teachers in those children." Mr. Shaw has lived about forty-six years in California and fifteen years in this home. The small free-standing duplex is in a neighborhood two blocks off busy San Pablo Avenue. During the late afternoon, prostitutes gather, dressed in fishnet stockings and short, tight leather skirts.

Inside the dimly lit living room is a very soiled carpet end serving as an area rug. A small coffee table is cluttered with plant cuttings. Mismatched furniture pieces are scattered in no apparent order by a window partially covered by ragged draperies. A rose-colored carved sofa, matching chair, and pink baroque ceramic lamps are placed at odd angles to the walls. What could be a dining room is piled high with assorted debris.

Albert says he moved to California to "better my condition." "I worked in a sawmill in Texas. The boss man would not let me work regular hours because I was black. I had a wife to support, never had children. I taught rural school, grades one through seven in Nacogdoches County. The principal taught grades seven through eleven. Rural school was all black and I enjoyed it but I had to stop at age thirty-nine when my eyes began to fail. I moved to California, along with everybody else, to work with the WPA as a tree cutter for the highways. Later, I worked with Uncle Sam—government jobs. When I was a young man I brought the mail, then graded lumber. I just sat there and the lumber rolled by and I marked it. I liked that job."

Retired for about sixteen or seventeen years, Mr. Shaw suffers from bad knees, diminished hearing, and near blindness. "I need all the help from all the sources. If I lay something down I can't find it."

A grocery store down the block delivers food and a sister-in-law next door cooks and does the laundry and cleaning. Albert's sister-in-law is eighty-nine herself and equally worn and ravaged by poverty. She lives with her daughter and checks in with Albert regularly. She is more physically fit than Albert but not at all satisfied with her advancing age.

Interestingly, Mr. Shaw's ex-wife lives just a few steps away, upstairs. They were married for about sixty years and when they divorced, the house was divided by a floor. He lives in five rooms downstairs and she lives in five rooms upstairs. Mrs. Shaw is eighty-one and is no longer a part of Albert's life.

Mr. Shaw enjoys numerous phone calls from church friends and a quick visit from a neighbor who delivers the mail. The mail carrier is a young man who thrusts his hand through the connecting door to the other duplex, expecting and finding Albert seated as usual on his straight-backed chair in the hallway. Albert has a great deal of difficulty opening the envelopes and he has no idea what is printed on the pages.

He has been trying to get on what he calls the "blind list" to receive some assistance with his disability. He has also been trying to get an appointment with his doctor for help to be declared blind. His physician has been serving the family for the past eight to ten years and practices in a medical complex in Oakland called "Pill Hill" by the locals. (The physician says Mr. Shaw had not been examined for nearly two years, and that he would have to be evaluated by an opthamologist in order to be declared blind. At my request, the physician called in the names and phone numbers of three local opthamologists. As of this writing, we are attempting to link Mr. Shaw with an opthamologist and arrange for the transportation and payment paperwork.)

Mr. Shaw says a church member calls occasionally to check in. A lady friend calls and brings covered dishes. "Seems like I'm pretty well thought of, but don't know if it's real," he says. "Everything that shines is not gold, you know."

Albert is pleased with his community, "This is a very nice settlement—peaceable—but I don't get out as much unless the deacons pick me up and take me to church."

Mr. Shaw says his major problem is money. There is simply not enough. He receives Social Security benefits and Navy retirement. His checks total about $400 a month. His utilities alone average $90 to $100 a month. When I asked if he was happy, Albert replied, "How can I be happy and broke?"

An average day begins when he leaves his bed, between 8 and 9 A.M. "At ninety-three, I take it easy now. I shower and have bacon and eggs. At 10:30 A.M. the van picks me up and I go to a meal site. I visit with people and have lunch. They bring me home between 1:30 and 2:00 P.M. Then I sit around and get bored. I can't see to read or watch TV. I listen to the radio [at full blast] and get phone calls."

It takes Mr. Shaw a long time to first hear, find, walk to, pick up, and answer the telephone. He says he does not get enough help when he needs it. He is careful not to add any complications to his life. "I don't fool with world affairs and ignore the bad eggs. I don't mess my hands up with bad people. What is important now is money and trying to get by."

Looking back over his life, Albert Shaw remembers two stories very clearly. The first is a bittersweet love affair with Callie, a young woman who lived on an adjacent farm in Texas. The second story is the long struggle to build Fulton Baxter Chapel Baptist Church in Oakland.

Albert recalls the lost love of Callie with such vivid sadness that their parting could have been days, not decades, ago. "When I was a very young man there was a girl who lived on a farm adjoining my daddy's farm. She was a pretty white girl—she sure was a pretty white girl. Callie and I grew up together and cared for one another. We met by an out-back fence and she told me, 'I wish that I was a colored girl or you a white boy—I'd take you.' I asked her if she wanted to get me killed! Our being caught together could get us killed. Callie is dead now. I learned awhile back that Callie had died."

Apparently Albert Shaw has enjoyed a relative amount of popularity with women. During the years that he worked for the U.S. mail service he had the attention of many women post office employees. "The white girls liked black men then and I liked them. I was thirty-five years old and healthy. There was discrimination with the U.S. mail and I could only work in the mail yard. One time I found twenty-two thousand dollars in checks in a sack. I knew how to cash them in but got the checks to the proper place. Funny, how I was kept out in the yard because I was black and then protected the nation's money. Maybe I should have kept the twenty-two thousand dollars."

The story of the Fulton Baxter Chapel Baptist Church is a long one that covers several years of Albert Shaw's life.

Fulton Baxter was an old man with a store-front church in Oakland. He and Albert had worked together in the WPA. Albert went to his church and liked his preaching. The little church was on Seventh Street in a tough neighborhood.

Albert Shaw, Fulton Baxter, and two other men decided to take on as their mission a project to create a larger, more proper church.

The men worked hard for six months and were able to save eleven hundred dollars in a bank account. This money became the down payment on an old house they wished to use as a church.

After Pearl Harbor, waves of workers moved to Oakland and the men were able to raise twenty-one hundred dollars, then nine thousand dollars and bought a larger stucco building. Albert petitioned to have the church named after his friend—the Fulton Baxter Chapel Baptist Church—and so it was.

Albert Shaw became a community leader and fund raiser.

After the congregation settled into the stucco building, Albert went to work and raised fifteen thousand dollars for a building fund. About that same time a Jewish synagogue went on sale in the real estate market for fifty thousand dollars. Mr. Shaw was put in charge of buying the building, if possible. It took three years. "Basically, it was a waiting game. I set up a building committee and we raised eleven thousand dollars in the bank. At the end of that same three years the price on the synagogue went down to thirty-five thousand dollars. We sold the stucco building for fifteen thousand dollars and added our eleven thousand dollars in the bank and bought the synagogue. You know, Fulton Baxter is an ugly old man, but a good preacher so we renamed the synagogue: Fulton Baxter Chapel Baptist Church."

It was only a matter of time before the chapel became too small. Church leaders looked at still another synagogue for sale where the avenues cross the streets in Oakland. This synagogue was also a large building and cost $565,000.

Albert felt like he was getting too old for this project and bowed out. "I can't perform the duties of a deacon now. Young stuff in there now can do it."

Mr. Shaw's younger counterparts have succeeded and they got the building and now it is almost paid for. Members crossing the threshold now enter the *Greater* Fulton Baxter Chapel Baptist Church!

Every time Albert goes to church on Sunday evening, they set a special dinner table for him in the pastor's study. He had dinner there two Sundays ago. He modestly acknowledges that he is treated with deference, respect, and affection.

Today, Mr. Shaw is entertaining himself with thoughts of looking for a wife. He does not regret never having had children. Given the state of the world, he says, "It's better not to have children." He wonders aloud and asks if he should marry again. He clearly has a lot to offer. He is thoughtful and affectionate. He has a long history of caring for others. He maintains a strong will and a glittering wit. Mr. Shaw reminded me as I left that, "We are all just passing through. We don't go this way but once. We have two roads to travel: one to destruction and one to life eternal—to live with God again."

Description and Analyses

Albert Shaw, near the end of his life, is an example of the fate of our very aged (those eighty-five and older) who find themselves with few monetary resources in a market economy.

What is different and new for Albert Shaw, as we approach the twenty-first century, is the very nature of the human life cycle itself, particularly in so-called developed nations that enjoy adequate or abundant resources and the blessings of hygeia. Specifically, significant and increasing numbers of human beings are spared the ravages of disease and violent death to live and ripen into a maturity of old—indeed venerable—age.

So, while a hallmark of successful human existence is our keen and speedy adaptability—albeit adaptation via culture—a lag exists between the ripple of change of increasing longevity being felt in every dimension of human group life, and our cultural adaptation to a graying of our population, particularly that segment of the aged at the end of the actuarial continuum—the old-old. Today, individuals entering the ranks of their eighth decade constitute the fastest-growing demographic trend in the United States.

Suzman and Riley (1985) place estimates of the eighty-five-plus age group at 2.6 million. Their numbers will also equal 5.2 percent of the population by the year 2050.

Data on the very aged are sparse and poorly understood. Suzman and Riley explain that although federal statistics are inadequate, a few trends are emerging. The picture unfolding of the old-old is they are very much like their younger counterparts, only more so. Patterns are accentuated. Suzman and Riley report the three major trends observed about the very aged is they are at the same time unique, heterogeneous, and changing. Very old members of the cohort are unique because they are predominantly female, less likely to be married, more likely to be living in an institution, and more likely to have little formal education. The very aged are also unique because they consume a disproportionate amount of public assistance.

The very aged are heterogeneous: while approximately 25 percent are institutionalized, the noninstitutionalized manage and function along a continuum. While 43 percent require personal assistance to carry out the activities of daily living, 57 percent function independently.

Finally, the very aged are constantly in a state of change. Structural flux

Table 10–1
Percentage distribution of age groups, by gender

Age Category	Female	Male
65–69	14.1	17.1
70–74	25.2	31.7
75–79	21.4	23.6
80–84	17.7	12.9
85–89	9.1	7.9
90+	12.4	6.7

is created as participation in one's eighth, ninth, or even tenth decade is exclusive and problematic. Social-psychological flux is created by a cohort effect in which the flow of each succeeding generation carries with it a shifting set of values, norms, and expectations.

Comparing these general patterns to the very aged participants in the California Senior Survey in table 10–1, we find 14.6 percent of men and 21.5 percent of women are eighty-five years old and older.

A demographic portrait of the oldest old developed by Rosenwaike (1985) reports 50 percent of the eighty-five-plus men as married, while only 8 percent of the women are still married. In addition, the dramatic shift in marital status for women occurs as they shift status from young-old (sixty-five to seventy-four) to old-old (eighty-five-plus). Rosenwaike's data count a majority (55 percent) of women married between the ages of sixty-five and sixty-nine, while a majority (82 percent) of those eight-five-plus are widowed.

Comparing these marital status figures to the CSS sample in table 10–2, the pattern continues. Between ages sixty-five and eighty-four, 62.5 percent of the CSS females were already widows and, at ages eighty-five and over, 76 percent widowed. A fractional 16.8 percent of the women sixty-five to

Table 10–2
Percentage distribution of marital status, by age group and gender

	Female		Male	
	Aged 65–84	Aged 85 +	Aged 65–84	Aged 85 +
	n=755	n=200	n=342	n=64
Marital Status	%	%	%	%
Married	16.8	8.5	48.5	53.1
Widowed	62.5	76.0	19.9	31.3
Single/Divorced	18.4	13.5	24.8	12.5
Separated	2.1	1.5	6.1	3.1
Other	0.1	0.5	0.6	0.0

Totals may not equal 100 percent exactly because of rounding.

eighty-four years old are married, while only half, or 8.5 percent, of the eighty-five-plus women still have a spouse. For men, marital status percentages are striking; 48.5 percent of those sixty-five to eighty-four years old are married and a larger proportion, 53.1 percent, of the eighty-five-plus group still has a living spouse.

In a sense, Albert Shaw exists in both these statistical worlds. Although he is divorced and separated by walls and floors, he still resides within the same household as his former wife.

However, in the statistical world of percentage distribution of the aged by ethnic status and age, Albert Shaw represents the rarest of the rare—the black man over ninety years old. There are only 2.9 percent of black men in the CSS plus-ninety age groups. This compares to the largest, 12.9 percent, for the plus-ninety Hispanic man group. If we count eighty-five-plus men by ethnic status, Albert Shaw's counterpart survivors still number the lowest, with 8.8 percent living. Table 10–3 data show the next largest surviving ethnic group is Asians at 13.5 percent, followed by whites at 15 percent and Hispanics at 25.8 percent.

Table 10–3 data also indicate the truly problematic time for black male longevity are years seventy to seventy-four, when they equal 38.2 percent of that age group. After age seventy-five the percent of black men falls dramatically.

Black women also fare the worst in their percentage distribution by age. Eighty-five-plus women represent 17.1 percent of the population, compared to 18.8 percent Asians, 22.3 percent whites, and 27.1 Hispanics.

The CSS population of black men eighty-five and older is only slightly older than the national percentage of 7.1 reported by Rosenwaike. Our greater share could in part be due to our sampling strategy, which selected Oakland for a sampling site expressly because of its large black population. On the other hand, Rosenwaike's data deal with the entire elderly population as a whole, whereas ours concern only the low income. It is reasonable to

Table 10–3
Percentage distribution of the CSS aged, by ethnic status and age group

Age Group	Female n=892				Male n=356			
	Asian %	Black %	Hisp %	White %	Asian %	Black %	Hisp %	White %
65–69	15.9	18.3	13.5	12.8	13.5	20.6	12.9	17.3
70–74	17.4	33.5	21.9	24.3	32.4	38.2	29.0	30.0
75–79	29.0	19.5	24.0	20.6	27.0	29.4	19.4	21.8
80–84	18.8	11.6	13.5	20.1	13.5	2.9	12.9	15.9
85–89	10.1	6.7	7.3	10.0	5.4	5.9	12.9	8.2
90+	8.7	10.4	19.8	12.3	8.1	2.9	12.9	6.8

Columns may not equal 100 percent because of rounding.

expect a greater percentage of black men among the low income given past patterns of economic discrimination.

Data in table 10–4, "Percentage distribution of noninstitutional living arrangements, by age group and gender," show Albert Shaw could again exist in two statistical columns. On the one side he is living very much alone, yet on the other side he resides in the same household as his former wife and they must share a common entry.

Living arrangements for the CSS aged are more easily defined because of the "forced-choice" questions, but Mr. Shaw's situation does point out potentials for interpretation problems involving in-law apartments with separate entries in R-1 rated neighborhoods. Granny flats and in-law apartments in R-1 neighborhoods have become so commonplace that Pacific Gas and Electric (the local utility company) routinely allows such households the lower kilowatt hour rate for a "multi-household" dwelling even though the in-law apartment arrangement is technically illegal and at variance with the zoning status.

Considering the number of elderly women who find themselves living alone, popularity of the in-law or granny flat and benign attitude of the utility company are timely indeed.

Well over 50 percent of all CSS females between sixty-five and eighty-four report living alone. A mere 13 percent of those sixty-five to eight-four years old continue to live with a spouse, while a fractional 6 percent of the eighty-five-and-over age group share a household with a husband.

For elderly men, living arrangement situations are the reverse—and more. Forty percent of men between sixty-five and eighty-four years old live alone, compared to 26.7 percent of those eighty-five and older. The compelling differences emerge on table 10–4 as one compares the relationship between gender and living with one's spouse. Thirty-three percent of men sixty-five to eighty-four years old reside with their spouses, while an impressive

Table 10–4
Percentage distribution of noninstitutional living arrangements, by age group and gender

Living Arrangements	Female		Male	
	Aged 65–84	Aged 85 +	Aged 65–84	Aged 85 +
Alone	57.7	54.5	40.2	26.7
With spouse	13.0	6.0	32.8	28.1
With children	9.6	17.5	2.4	12.5
With spouse and children	1.9	0.5	9.7	9.4
With children and grandchldrn.	5.6	2.0	1.5	0.0
With siblings	2.7	1.7	0.9	2.9
Board & care	1.8	2.0	0.9	3.1
Other[a]	8.6	14.0	8.4	17.1

[a]"Other" includes living with other relatives, with nonrelatives, with paid provider, etc.

28.1 percent of the post-eighty-five men do too. This is nearly five times more than women of the eighty-five-and-over group.

A second compelling statistic is the comparative number of women who shared a household with children or grandchildren. While 5.6 percent of women sixty-five to eighty-four live with children and grandchildren, only 1.5 percent of the men do. And, for the eighty-five-plus group, 2 percent of women reside with offspring, while no men were reported in that category. This finding may be a product of differential longevity, machismo, or lifelong patterns of family relations such as the preference for "intimacy at a distance" noted in chapter 4. Particularly for CSS participants, a living situation with children and grandchildren may be a matter of economic necessity. Given patterns of differential longevity, poor women are more likely to outlive their sparse resources.

Although CSS women may live longer, they do not enjoy better health during the added lifetime. Self-report health status for the sixty-five- to eighty-four-years-old age group in table 10–5 finds nearly equal percentages of men and women report good, fair, and poor health. However, in all three response categories, it is the men who report being slightly healthier. Thirty-nine percent of men report "good" health, compared to 38 percent of women. Both men and women have an equivalent "fair" health status at 45.5 and 45.6 percent respectively. Finally, "poor" health is endured by 15.2 percent of the men, compared to 16.3 percent of the women.

Curiously, comparative health status of women goes into a sharp decline in the very aged group. Fifty-three percent of men report "good" health, compared to 38 percent of women. Percentages balance out in the middle category with 39.1 percent of men and 47.5 percent of women reporting "fair" health. The surprising dip comes in the last category where approximately twice as many women report "poor" health: 14.1 and 7.8 percent, respectively.

For CSS participants, this apparent declining health of women may be a function of underreporting by men; survival of the fittest of the men; or perceived poorer health on the part of women. There is accumulating evidence

Table 10–5
Percentage distribution of self-reported health
status, by age group and gender

	Aged 65–84		Aged 85+	
	Female	*Male*	*Female*	*Male*
Health	$n=748$	$n=342$	$n=198$	$n=64$
Status	%	%	%	%
Good	38.2	39.2	38.4	53.1
Fair	45.5	45.6	47.5	39.1
Poor	16.3	15.2	14.1	7.8

in the women's studies literature that all women, particularly poor women, including homemakers, engage in enormous amounts of unreported, unrecognized, and unpaid labor. Working poor women with families often labor the equivalent of two full-time jobs (Steinem 1983).

The superior health status of very aged men is further specified in table 10–6, "Independent physical functioning in Activities of Daily Living." In the sixty-five- to eighty-four-years-old age category, men and women only differ by three percentage points in areas of bathing, dressing, toileting, incontinence, transfer, and eating.

Again, in the post-eighty-five age group, more men were independent than women in every single activity. Between 90.6 and 98.4 percent of the post-eighty-five males were independent in all six activities.

As a group, the very aged are relatively independent in their activities of daily living. With the one exception—albeit an important one—of incontinence in post-eighty-five females, at least 80 percent of all CSS participants independently manage bathing, dressing, toileting, transfer, and eating.

The picture of independent functioning is significantly different for the Instrumental Activities of Daily Living.

Table 10–7 data show that in movement outside the house, like shopping and travel, independence drops off sharply.

Of interest is a continuing poorer physical functioning in the Instrumental Activities of Daily Living for very old women. In seven of the eight IADL categories men eighty-five and older scored higher percentages of instrumental independence. Men score within a range of 49.2 percent independent for shopping to 88.2 percent independent for medications.

Telephoning is the only activity where women score a higher 88.5 percent independent, compared to 82.8 percent for men. Our speculation about this difference suggests perhaps all those years of women's affective, nurturing and contact behaviors—including electronic contacts—paid off. Women used the telephone frequently and did not lose the skill. This, however, does

Table 10–6
Percentage distribution of independent physical functioning in Activities of Daily Living, by age group and gender

	Female		Male	
	Aged 65–84	Aged 85+	Aged 65–84	Aged 85+
	n=747	n=200	n=341	n=64
Activitiy	%	%	%	%
Bathing	89.0	80.0	88.9	90.6
Dressing	95.5	88.5	94.7	95.3
Toileting	96.7	93.0	95.9	96.9
Incontinence	83.2	73.0	86.8	92.2
Transfer	95.7	91.0	97.1	95.3
Eating	99.2	96.0	98.8	98.4

Table 10–7
Percentage distribution of independent physical functioning in Instrumental
Activities of Daily Living, by age group and gender

	Female		Male	
	Aged 65–84 *n=747*	*Aged 85+* *n=200*	*Aged 65–84* *n=340*	*Aged 85+* *n=64*
Activity	*%*	*%*	*%*	*%*
Shopping	47.0	30.2	54.1	49.2
Travel	53.0	33.5	71.6	68.8
Medications	91.4	80.8	85.0	88.2
Telephoning	93.6	88.5	92.4	82.8
Money Mgt.	89.9	76.4	85.6	81.3
Laundry	77.5	56.5	71.8	61.5
Food Preparation	74.8	61.4	64.0	66.7
Housework	80.1	67.7	80.1	73.1

not explain why women scored less independent than males in such traditional female activities as shopping, laundry, food preparation, and housework.

We believe, on the one hand, men who survive to eighty-five or older are
a cultural and biological elite; on the other hand, women in their eighth decade may be a gender elite but individually exhausted. Clearly, more study is
needed about the paid and unpaid work of women and the long-term effects
of these labors on their functional independence during the aging process.

For the nearly 30 percent women and 20 percent men who are intellectu-
ally impaired, the likelihood of potential informal support candidates, described in table 10–8, is critical. For the very aged, living children able to
provide ongoing care is relatively problematic. The eighty-five-year-old
woman who bore a child at age twenty has a young-old potential caregiver
now sixty-five.

Among the CSS sample, 22 percent of the women and 30 percent of the
men reported no living children. By the time individuals reach their eighth

Table 10–8
Percentage distribution of number of living children among the CSS very
old, by gender (22 percent of the females and 30 percent of the males
reported no living children)

Number of *Children*	*Female*	*Male*	*Mean Number* *of Children* *for Category*
1–2	53.6	37.8	1.49
3–5	35.5	35.6	3.69
6–8	8.4	17.8	6.67
More than 8	2.6	8.9	10.25

decade, they have outlived most of their peers, and the actuarial tables have taken a toll on their children.

Table 10–8 data reveal approximately 75 percent of very aged who still have living children. The mean number of 53.6 percent of the women and 37.8 percent of the men is 1.49. The next highest category is three to five children, with a mean of 3.69 for 35.5 percent of women and 35.6 percent of men.

As we have reported in chapter 4 and elsewhere (Clark and Pelham 1982; 1983), these children are actively involved in organizing and providing informal support for their elder parents. Questions remaining open, however, involve individuals like Albert Shaw who have no children for biological reasons; individuals who choose not to have children for life-style reasons, such as lesbians and gays; and individuals whose children are becoming aged themselves. For example, we know of three older sons who wish to provide needed labor for frail mothers and an aunt. All three sons are limited because of poor health. One son has since died of coronary artery disease.

Personal and social costs of providing informal support and the dimensions of younger or older care providers remains poorly understood.

In Albert Shaw's case, his only personal care comes from a visibly worn sister-in-law who is eighty-nine years old. His care is poor at best and we can only wonder at her costs of working for a man who is not even a blood relative.

The second line of defense for support needs are grandchildren. Very aged participants in the CSS report 28 percent of women and 30 percent of men had no living grandchildren.

These percentages are roughly equal to the numbers of CSS participants who have no living children. In table 10–9, for those who have grandchildren, mean numbers are slightly higher than for children, with an increasing percentage of the very aged having more grandchildren after the fifth grandchild. This stands to reason as the longer a child lives, the more likelihood

Table 10–9
Percentage distribution of the number of living grandchildren among the CSS very old, by gender (28 percent of the females and 30 percent of the males reported no living grandchildren)

Number of Grandchildren	Female	Male	Mean Number of Grandchildren for Category
1–2	21.4	20.0	1.61
3–5	29.7	31.1	3.98
6–8	13.1	17.8	6.96
More than 8	35.8	31.1	16.41

Table 10–10
Percentage distribution of living siblings among the CSS very old, by
gender (45 percent of the females and 34 percent of the males report no
living siblings)

Number of Siblings	Female	Male	Mean Number of Siblings for Category
1–2	63.1	62.8	1.42
3–5	30.7	27.9	3.74
6–8	4.4	9.3	6.56
More than 8	1.8	0.0	9.00

he or she is to produce offspring, particularly career women who may delay
childbearing until their late thirties or early forties. A woman who bears a
child at forty and whose daughter herself bears a child at forty will not be a
grandmother until age eighty. Long-range demographic and social consequences of the reproduction biological clock ticking away for baby boom
career women who are now approaching forty remain to be seen. If the off-
spring is male, however, and, given that men tend to marry women who are
younger, "grandmotherhood" would more likely occur in the seventh decade.

A circle of informal support is often made stronger by involvement of
siblings. Table 10–10 outlines by gender the percentage distribution of living
siblings among the very old.

By the time an individual has reached eighty-five he or she has lost many
birth family members. Forty-five percent of women and 34 percent of men
have no living siblings.

For the very aged with siblings fortunate enough to inherit a long-lived
gene pool, about 63 percent of both men and women still have one to two
living brothers or sisters, with a mean number of 1.42.

As we reported in chapter 4 and elsewhere, contact between the aged
and their children is relatively frequent. Table 10–11 data indicate women

Table 10–11
Percentage distribution of the frequency of contact of young-old and old-
old with children, by gender

Frequency of Contact	Aged 65–84		Aged 85+	
	Female	Male	Female	Male
Today, yesterday	61.43	53.04	67.60	62.79
2–7 days ago	24.64	22.17	23.80	20.93
8–30 days ago	7.50	9.57	5.30	6.98
Over a month ago	6.43	15.22	3.31	9.30

receive the most contact in both the young-old and the old-old categories. In a seven-day period, 86 percent of the women sixty-five to eighty-four and 91 percent of the women eighty-five-plus have had contact with a child. Men are only somewhat lower, 75 and 83 percent respectively. If the time frame is increased to one month, contact in each age and gender group tops 90 percent, except in the young-old men at 84 percent.

Table 10–12 data show frequency of contact with women continues as percentage distributions of contacts with siblings remain relatively constant over the years.

Approximately 44 percent of the sixty-five- to eighty-four-years-old and very aged women age groups have had contact with a brother or sister during the past seven days. Likewise, approximately 30 percent of men sixty-five to eighty-four years old and eighty-five-plus have either seen or heard from a sibling during the past week.

Supportive tasks for a young-old or old-old individual can be as intimate as bathing or instrumental as home repairs. Table 10–13 lists twenty tasks of daily living support reported by CSS participants. General patterns show needs for assistance are greater for instrumental activities (e.g., shopping and housework) and less so for personal care (e.g., toileting and transfer).

A cross-check of the columns indicates that, in almost every single cell, for twenty tasks, man or women, young-old or old-old, the larger percentage of care is provided by the informal support system. The one individual exception by three percentage points is "housework," provided to eighty-five-plus women by the formal system. The one general exception is "home repairs," where larger percentages are uniformly provided by formal support. In this case the formal support provider is the landlord.

Albert Shaw follows a parallel pattern of an intersection between informal and formal support. He can feed, dress, and bathe himself without assistance. Formal support enters his life at out-of-doors instrumental activities. Mr. Shaw requires accompanying and transport for a prepared meal and some social network contact.

We believe Albert Shaw requires still more formal support to improve the quality of this existence. Clearly feeble attempts by his sister-in-law re-

Table 10–12

Percentage distribution of the frequency of contact of young-old and old-old with siblings, by gender

Frequency of Contact	Aged 65–84		Aged 85 +	
	Female	*Male*	*Female*	*Male*
Today, yesterday	22.51	10.87	19.44	21.43
2–7 days ago	21.51	19.57	24.07	9.52
8–30 days ago	16.53	13.91	12.04	16.67
Over a month ago	39.44	55.65	44.94	52.38

Table 10–13
Percentage distribution of formal and informal support reported by the young-old and old-old, by gender

| Tasks | Aged 85 + | | | | Aged 65–84 | | | |
| | Male (332) | | Female (731) | | Male (64) | | Female (198) | |
	Inf.	Form.	Inf.	Form.	Inf.	Form.	Inf.	Form.
Toileting	3	1	2	1	3	0	7	1
Dressing	4	1	4	2	5	0	11	7
Transfer	2	≤1	2	1	3	2	8	3
Bathing	9	3	7	5	9	2	13	11
Eating/Feeding	2	1	2	1	8	0	5	4
Walking	4	2	4	2	3	0	10	4
Outside mobility	7	2	14	5	8	0	24	10
Wheelchair use	2	≤1	1	1	2	0	5	4
Stair climbing	3	1	6	2	3	2	9	2
Laundry	34	14	23	15	36	19	30	25
Telephone	6	2	8	1	13	0	11	5
Money Mgt.	20	2	19	2	19	5	34	5
Travel	17	5	31	7	23	3	43	10
Shopping	31	8	40	10	39	8	47	21
Housework	34	13	20	18	38	20	27	30
Medicine	8	3	5	2	5	3	12	7
Meal prep.	32	10	13	9	38	9	19	18
Social network	14	1	21	2	16	2	29	5
Home repairs	8	32	19	34	14	25	22	35
Accompanying (official visits)	4	5	25	7	22	2	27	9

quire and deserve some relief. Mr. Shaw needs assistance with outside mobility, stair climbing, laundry, money management, travel, shopping, housework, taking his medications, meal preparation, social network, and home repairs. He also needs medical attention. A problematic informal system is inadequate, fragile, and strained.

The question of who is helping is equally important to what tasks are being done.

Although most CSS respondents do not report a need for assistance, for those who do, their needs are being met by women—wives and daughters. These findings confirm a virtual mountain of data on the enormous amount of informal support provided to the aged (mostly women) by women (table 10–14).

Medical Expenditures

To place the very aged in a larger social context of relationships to larger social systems, we examine their relative consumption of Medicare and Medicaid dollars.

Table 10–14
Modal providers of informal support to the CSS very old, by gender and marital status

| | Female | | Male | |
Tasks	Married $n=5$	Spouseless $n=145$	Married $n=8$	Spouseless $n=30$
Meals	Spouse, Son, Child-in-Law (Trimodal)	Daughter	Spouse	Daughter
Laundry	Child-in-Law	Daughter	Spouse	Daughter
Walking	Son	Daughter	Spouse	Daughter
Walking with aids	Son, Child-in-Law	Daughter	None	Daughter
Stairs	Son	Daughter	None	Son
Telephone	None	Daughter	Spouse	Daughter
Grooming	Son	Daughter	Spouse	Daughter
Feeding	Son	Daughter	Spouse	Daughter
Foot care	Spouse, Son	Daughter	Spouse	Daughter
Housework	Son, Daughter	Daughter	Spouse	Daughter
Dressing	Son	Daughter	Spouse	Daughter
Bathing	Son	Daughter	Spouse	Daughter
Toileting	Son	Daughter	None	None
Money	Son	Daughter	Spouse	Daughter
Shopping	Son, Daughter	Daughter	Spouse	Daughter

The array of percentages on table 10–15 displays vividly that even the very aged poor are responsible for fewer expenditures than their younger counterparts.

For the highest average monthly claim of five hundred dollars and over, the eighty-five-plus age group is consuming less than half, 11.2 percent, than their younger counterparts, at 23 percent.

Further, for the plus-ninety age group, percentages of expenditures for Medicare claims are less in seven of the eleven dollar categories.

Average monthly paid claims for Medicaid mirror expenditures of Medicare. Table 10–16 shows that for the highest average monthly claim of five hundred dollars and over, consumption of public dollars is lower.

While the difference in percent of expenditures is only fractional—two-tenths of one percent—between the groups sixty-five to eighty-four years old and eighty-five-plus, that fact is telling. Only 6.1 percent of the eighty-five-plus age group had Medicaid claims of five hundred dollars and over, compared to 6.3 percent for the sixty-five- to eighty-four-years-old age category. The very aged CSS participants are not claiming a larger or disproportionate amount of Medicaid or Medicare.

Table 10–15
Percentage distribution of average monthly Medicare
expenditures, by age group

Average Monthly Paid Claims	65–69	70–74	75–79	80–84	85–89	90+
$0–$49	80.8	73.6	75.7	73.1	71.7	82.3
$50–$99	6.2	6.4	4.9	7.0	9.4	6.9
$100–$149	1.6	5.5	3.0	3.2	3.8	1.5
$150–$199	2.1	1.8	2.7	1.6	3.8	1.5
$200–$249	0.5	1.8	1.9	3.2	0.9	0.0
$250–$299	0.5	1.2	1.9	1.1	0.9	1.5
$300–$349	0.0	1.2	1.9	0.5	0.0	0.8
$350–$499	0.0	0.6	1.1	1.1	1.9	0.0
$400–$449	2.1	0.9	1.1	1.6	0.9	0.8
$450–$499	1.0	1.2	0.4	0.5	0.0	0.0
$500+	5.2	5.5	5.3	7.0	6.6	4.6

Perhaps more important is that the poor aged as a group are not found at the high end of average monthly paid Medicaid claims.

For the very aged, 84.9 percent of the eighty-five-plus group and 88.5 percent of the ninety-plus group have average monthly claims of less than one hundred dollars.

Incredibly, in the ninety-plus age group, Medicaid expenditures are zero in five of the eleven categories. This finding correlates with the situation of Albert Shaw, who had not seen a physician in years.

Table 10–16
Percentage distribution of average monthly Medi-Cal
(Medicaid) expenditures, by age groups

Average Monthly Paid Claims	65–69	70–74	75–79	80–84	85–89	90+
$0–$49	65.8	61.0	61.6	64.5	59.4	65.4
$50–$99	21.2	21.8	22.4	21.0	25.5	23.1
$100–$149	7.3	7.7	8.8	5.9	5.7	3.1
$150–$199	2.6	3.4	2.7	2.7	1.9	5.4
$200–$249	0.5	3.1	1.1	2.7	1.9	0.0
$250–$299	0.0	0.3	1.1	0.0	0.0	0.0
$300–$349	0.5	0.6	0.8	1.1	0.9	0.0
$350–$499	0.0	0.0	0.0	0.0	0.9	0.0
$400–$449	0.0	0.3	0.4	0.5	0.0	0.0
$450–$499	0.0	0.3	0.0	0.0	0.0	0.8
$500+	2.1	1.5	1.1	1.6	3.8	2.3

11
Theoretical Considerations

Paradigm Problems

Behavioral and social science theorists, like all theorists, are in the business of explaining and predicting phenomena. Explaining and predicting human aging phenomena is complicated by the multitude of disciplines—and analytic frameworks within each discipline—that attempt to envision a better understanding of aging.

As aging is at the same time a biological, psychological, social, and even spiritual phenomenon, it is necessary for the theories we weave to be interdisciplinary. A truly global theory of aging will not exist until we can meld all dimensions of aging into a comprehensive and coherent structure and finally arrive at the realization that theories are socially constructed. Theories are products of culture, language, history, methodologies, social class, domain assumptions, and personal sentiments. In short, theories are very human creations.

Herein lies the paradigm problem. To set the foundation for our exploration of aging theory, we must digress briefly into the realms of philosophy and epistemology.

Our beliefs about the nature of human knowledge (and the subset of theory) are grounded in the traditions of the sociology of knowledge; a tradition that posits that human knowledge (whether scientific or everyday) is socially created, socially distributed, and, in a very real sense, is a commodity. Knowledge, like other commodities, is linked to social structures, social class, and power. As such, what is taken for granted as "objective truth" is actually truth according to interest groups who identify, segment, and define truth and have the power to enforce definitions. Joan of Arc is an example of a short-term loser in a battle over the generation and distribution—indeed power—to control sacred knowledge.

Epistemological work of Marx, Mannheim, Gouldner, Kuhn, and Berger and Luckman profoundly shape our analytics. A common thread in their analyses is that there is no such entity as an *a priori* reality "out there"—

outside of our minds—to somehow observe, test, measure, understand, explain, and predict. External phenomena are comprehended only in relation to internal learned comprehension. A cup of red wine does not exist *a priori* in nature for the scholar to interpret. A cup is a unit of measure, red is a color, wine is a human-made beverage both sacred and profane. Wine is a word that conjures up meaning, beliefs, and values. Thus, enologists, like gerontologists, enter life's vineyards with a multitude of sociocultural analytic grids already in place.

Specifically, our *Weltanschauung* says: economic substructures fundamentally affect societal superstructures and ideology; ideas, beliefs, values, everyday and scientific knowledge—including theories—are embedded in social structures; all scientific theories contain a set of implicit "background assumptions" that are theorists' internalized sociocultural constructs; reality, including the assumed "*a priori* objectivity" of scientific theory is *not*. Paradigms are socially constructed. Paradigms are *not* independent of human experience and interest, as the following recapitulation and critique illustrates.

This problem is a difficult one indeed because we are reminded that what we experience and know and believe depends upon the structure of our senses, minds, cultures, class, and paradigms. Our eye cannot see infra-red or ultra-violet ends of the light spectrum, but who will deny these lights/colors exist? They exist because we identify and define their natures. We have made them real. This is the problem of the instrument attempting to measure itself, Plato's shadows on the cave wall, blind men describing an elelphant, or the physicist attempting to push the bus upon which she is riding. Even given these limitations to knowledge, this mind set of epistemological assumptions leads us to adopt a framework that at the macro level focuses upon the *political economy* of aging, and, at the micro level, focuses upon *symbolic interactionism*, that is, the process of meaning arising from interpretation and interaction in human groups.

Both levels are necessary, because without a macro-level analysis we ignore the larger social and economic forces that influence the trajectories of individual lives. For example, without an understanding of the sex discrimination that exists in the labor markets, which we discussed in chapter 1, we will not fully understand the relatively greater incidence of poverty among elderly women. Conversely, a macro analysis without micro-level analysis, particularly when using the methods and frameworks of symbolic interactionism, misses hearing and understanding the voices of the major participants—the aged poor—as they speak.

So what is our solution? We conceptualize these frameworks reflecting off one another like a hall of mirrors. For example, at the macro level, interest-group politics generates personal aging troubles, patterns of personal aging troubles create interest-group politics (with varying degrees of power, of course). Likewise, at the micro level, individuals perceive, interact, give meaning to, modify through an interpretative process, adapt to (or not), and change the phenomena of human aging, and the social constructions of it. Individual life chances, experiences, or troubles have only relative relationships to personality, adaptive skills, or pathology. Individual life trajectories are inextricably linked to social class, social structures, and socioeconomic forces. We must have a self-awareness of the social creation and analytic construction of human aging and an acknowledgment of the implicit, even sometimes "subconscious," assumptions and ideology inherent in all aging theory. Grandmothers, geezers, and gomers were not created by the gods on Olympus. Socio/economic/political structures and ideologies create and are themselves created by and in human groups.

However, we cannot, in this present work, adequately present the type of structural analysis this topic merits and we concentrate more on the micro, individual level while acknowledging the need for more macro analyses. The work of Minkler and Estes (1984) goes a long way in this direction.

What we learned about the old and poor from our study and the vignettes is relatively simple. Many of the poor aged were low income or near poor for most of their lives. Retirement and accumulating deficits (e.g., a lifetime of inadequate nutrition and health care, little education, no savings, poor housing, and transportation) add up to tip the balance into poverty, a still lower quality of life, human suffering, and death. The prevalence of such negative outcomes are much greater among women and minorities. What the aged poor need, given the present level of access to medical care, is simply more money to allay their worries about "Social Insecurity" and how they are going to make it through the end of the month on less than five hundred dollars.

Money does indeed purchase life's cornucopia. And that is the *major difference* between the poor and affluent elderly—money and the opportunities and alternatives it represents. Economics literally affect the trajectory of the aging process and experience. The cumulative effect of lifelong near-poverty shows up most dramatically in the morbidity and mortality rates of the aged poor. At the same time, there are those who blame the aged poor for their higher rates of medical expenditures and would want to make them scapegoats when discussing national fiscal and budgetary priorities.

As we will see in the ensuing discussion, aging theory is still operating, for the most part, at the level of jousting analytic frameworks. Never mind paradigm wars.

Traditions of Aging Theory

Groundwork for a structure of aging theory began in the mid-fifties and early sixties. The tradition of aging theory is posited in two formal sociological analyses that attempt to explain and predict aging phenomena: the activity theory (Havighurst and Albrecht 1953) and the polar opposite disengagement theory (Cumming and Henry 1961). Briefly stated, activity theory assumes that the relationship between the individual and society remains relatively stable over time. The aging individual is allowed to "slow down a little," but since affecting norms are essentially the same as in midlife, he or she is expected to make the necessary adjustments. As roles diminish and losses increase, elders are obliged to compensate by adding roles and extending activities. The man or woman's continuing life satisfaction depends upon keeping active. The basic postulates of activity theory are:

P1 The greater the loss, the less activity one is likely to engage in.
P2 The greater the activity, the more role support one is likely to receive.
P3 The more role support one receives, the more positive one's self-concept is likely to be.
P4 The more positive one's self-concept, the greater one's satisfaction is likely to be.

Disengagement theory, on the other hand, assumes exactly the contrary. It postulates that the essential, necessary, and natural relationship between an aging individual and society is one of mutual withdrawal. The process is both social and psychological. This relationship functions to free the weakening individual for satisfying introspection as death draws near and simultaneously enables society to prepare for the ultimate loss of the individual.

Critique of Assumptions of the Tradition

When activity and disengagement theories are compared to the aging experience of poor elders, their explanatory and predictive powers have serious problems and flaws.

Disengagement theory simply does not account for the data. It neither predicts nor explains interaction processes and variations in adaptation, such as the newly arrived individuals in the San Francisco Tenderloin hotels learning how to get a free meal in a new culture. Empirically speaking, disengagement has not occurred for the vast majority of the poor elderly, even though many are quite old and living in a social environment that is sometimes withdrawing and hostile. While it is true that a small proportion of the aged poor have retired to a reclusive existence, we must ask why and under what conditions and understand that most have not. For example, our most reclusive subject, Mr. Shaw, was confined to his walker because of chronic health problems rather than a desire to spend the day sitting in the hallway. Also, as he pointed out, it takes money to enjoy yourself these days. His experience indicates that withdrawal is more a function of economic class, medical phenomena, and environment than an instinctual action. Disengagement for Mr. Shaw is more accurately a forced status he has little power to resist. Finally, even with his problems, Mr. Shaw made it out every day to the congregate meal center, and he hungers for human companionship. If anything, most elderly individuals seem more aware of their environment and their relationship to it than counterparts in youth and mid-life.

If aging is the independent variable and the disengagement is the dependent variable, then the logic of the theory is faulty. This flaw can be corrected as Hochschild (1975) suggests, by making disengagement a variable process rather than a static occurrence. One could argue that at some point some form of disengagement will occur—if only for a few seconds before death.

Whether disengagement is universal, inevitable, and intrinsic is no longer a subject of active debate. The evidence continually argues that disengagement theory is no longer a valid conceptual construct that merits further testing. The question of universality depends upon the assumed definition of successful aging; the question of intrinsic biological reduction and inevitability requires empirical validation which is impossible to provide because one cannot separate out the effects of the environment and social policies on behaviors which may appear to be disengagement-like. What we have seen is that individuals, *in spite of environmental effects and social policies,* will still struggle to participate in the everyday commerce of life.

According to our findings among the aged poor, the three propositions of disengagement theory—universal, inevitable, and intrinsic—prove false. A willed disengagement is neither characteristic nor common among the aged poor. It is neither inherent in the vast majority of old-old and dying nor singly caused by biological forces.

The four stated postulates of activity theory fare a little better when compared to our study. However, it is important to remember that the postulates relate activity theory to life satisfaction. Disengagement theory principally attempts to answer the question "What is aging?" with the assumption that successful aging means mutual withdrawal, while activity theory asks, "What constitutes successful aging?"

Comparing the activity theory postulates with our data, we find that diminishing activity does not necessarily follow a loss of roles. In fact, often the opposite is true. Individuals create new and complex roles, and in the process of acting them out, consume enormous amounts of time.

Whether one receives role support for a particular activity depends upon the role and the activity.

Many individuals remain symbolically active in former and current worlds and participate technologically via radio and television. Individuals reinforce their own self-concepts. What is important is the individual's construction of reality, the meanings that are attached to experience.

It is the nature of the role and the meaning attached to it that is critical. Linking positive self-concept and role support assumes that the role is a positive one and reinforced. However, one might enjoy a positive self-concept from a so-called negative role (e.g., "crafty drug pusher" or "loan shark"). It also presumes that self-concept is entirely dependent upon the performance of a role, and that all behavior is role behavior. For example, the Tenderloin hotel "pest" receives support for his "pest" role, but his self-esteem, self-concept, and life satisfaction are relatively low. In contrast, the former journalist, who lives today on memories, enjoys high self-esteem even though there is a minute amount or even absence of role support. To say that a positive self-concept is related to greater life satisfaction is tautology. For this to be true for the aged poor, one would have to ask "under what conditions?" This question should be asked partly in order to address the problem of power. The issue of power is for the most part overlooked by activity theory and by disengagement theory as well.

Whether disengagement is universal, inevitable, and intrinsic remains to be seen. The question of universality awaits cross-cultural comparisons; the question of inevitability depends upon the assumed definition of successful aging, and the question of intrinsic biological reduction requires empirical validation and is also philosophically debatable.

Perhaps the most serious flaw in both activity and disengagement theories is the omission of *meaning*. Both theories have been constructed in a phenomenological and ethnomethodological desert where an actor's interpretation of reality and the social determinants that shape it are neglected. This difficulty is posited, first, in philosophical assumptions about the nature of scientific theory (a paradigm problem), and second, in philosophical assumptions about the nature of humankind. This paradigm problem rests in the structure of scientific activity, where social scientific paradigms are forced onto the process of growing old, like procrustean cookie cutters on rolled dough. To balance, a phenomenological analysis says that the enterprise should be more the other way around. First there needs to be a distinction made between aging as a biological process and growing old as a social process. Second, the "rolled dough" of the *social construction* of growing old should be left whole, carefully observed, and allowed to emerge into whatever it may be with the assistance of a phenomenological procrustean cookie cutter. That is, study the meanings of social action for actors. Morris (1977) explains:

> Such a study would not begin by imposing a theory upon the phenomenon of aging but instead would explore the ways in which all aspects of age are talked about, depicted in the media of mass communication, lived, endured and enjoyed, used, negotiated, and changed from day to day.

Growing old is a very complex and still largely unknown phenomenon. It is a jumble of biological, psychological, sociological, cultural, and historical realities. It is not an objective phenomenon existing outside our consciousness. We are forced to choose among "procrustean cookie cutters" where giving meaning to our existence is concerned. We do not simply stumble upon meanings already assigned by a god or nature or a cosmetics company.

The "nature of humankind" problem is an old one and to a great degree it is a paradigm problem as well. It seems clear that any theory that hopes to explain human group life yet fails to take into account the socially reflexive nature of humans—meanings derived by social interaction and modified over time—is somewhat incomplete.

Until all levels of reality are addressed in a single theory or accounted for in a comprehensive collection of analytic frameworks, the impediments to formal aging theory will remain. For example, so-called life satisfaction and depression scales measure an individual's reaction to a social situation(s). If the individual is dissatisfied or depressed, s/he is labeled as "adapting poorly," has "mental health problems," or, worse yet, is "pathological." Never mind how they got that way. Nowhere are such scales and indices questioning the legitimacy or reasonableness of responses. One supposes it to be perfectly normal to feel depressed about a forced retirement, a dramatic reduction in income, difficulty locating affordable housing, and a problematic health care system.

The larger questions are rarely asked: under what conditions do individuals have low scores in life statisfaction and depression scales?; who really benefits from producing a particular social situation or condition?; or whose interests are served by the creation of community problems?

A more comprehensive approach might start out by inquiring how individual troubles (and successes) in aging are connected to larger social structures, how these same structures create and are supported by ideology, and how all of these taken together maintain (or question) the social order.

Role, Stratification, and Subcultural Frameworks

In addition to the activity and disengagement theories, there are a number of theoretical approaches to social aging that strive to test and explain theoretical categories and concepts, for example, role, stratification, and subculture.

Role

Phillips (1957), Rosow (1974), and others have long argued that role theory can go a long way toward answering the question, "What happens to human beings socially as they grow old?" In this analysis, generally speaking, social roles are seen as independent variables, and adjustment in old age, including self-conceptions, are viewed as dependent variables.

Phillips' framework attempts to predict the degree of adjustment of the aged. The equation is delineated by the concept of "age identification" as an intervening variable between each role change and adjustment. Although Phillips' clarification inserts the element of individual perception, relationships between the variables remain unclear and the variables themselves are, at the same time, speculative in definition and crude in application. The "role as causal" analytic framework views only one narrow band of reality. An analysis of the structures and functions of social roles leaves out the process of creating meanings regarding those roles; it fails to consider the conditions under which new roles are, or are not, created; it overlooks all other behaviors not related to role performance; and, finally, it assumes that social structures are more important than social processes in explaining the aging experience. That is, the social construction of the reality of aging as a dialectic process is absent from the analysis.

Rosow (1974) conceptualizes aging as a transition into a roleless, normless state that is qualitatively different from middle age. The reason for the dysfunction is the absence of structures that function to facilitate socialization to old age. Rosow argues that old age "tends top develop gradually and informally" with "few public observances of a status change."

Second, Rosow contends that "there is a severe alienation from central social roles," "a loss of rewards," "a mounting curve of illness and physical handicap," and "correlates of dependency, isolation, and demoralization."

Third, Rosow supposes that "old age is marked by sharp role discontinuity, especially for men. . . . For women, the transition is usually not so abrupt. . . . Women can adapt to their declining role more slowly, in less abrupt stages."

Stratification

The second analytic framework also focuses on social structures, but at a societal level. It is the age stratification analysis developed by Riley (1971). The macro-level orientation of this theory views social class as a multidimensional independent variable affecting both the individual experience and the social dynamics of aging. It asks how social class affects an individual's attitudes on aging and concomitant behavior; how social class influences relationships between and within age strata; what difficulties face upwardly or downwardly mobile individuals; and finally, what the ramifications are of age strata and social class for a change in the larger society. The age statification analysis assumes the existence of social class and age strata as relative givens, and asks rather how social order is created given structural con-straints and problematic interactional processes.

The four broad areas of inquiry outlined by Riley are intriguing when compared to the social worlds of the aged poor. For example, attitudes and certainly behaviors differ widely among and between social strata of the aged. Social class is an important variable to be sure, but not sufficient in the causal sense of affecting change by itself. An illustration is the fact that a number of aged individuals who are highly educated, former professionals, and economically comfortable enough to do otherwise—choose to live in the inner city. Clearly they have a set of life-style priorities not neatly predicted by their social class. Second, although social class influences on relationships between and within age strata are not the focus of this research, our observa-tions suggest that no real differences exist in the quality and quantity of social contacts among and between the aged poor and their affluent counterparts. That is, while controlling for social context, the numbers and kinds of social contacts by friends and relatives appear to be approximately equal. Many of the affluent aged are lonely too. Third, downward mobility is a much more complex process than many suppose and it does not always necessarily imply a totally negative change. We have observed numbers of aged women "blooming" after divorce or the death of a dominating husband, even though it also meant a step down the economic ladder and the loss of one social role and status.

Perhaps Rose (1965) can be some help in deciphering that apparent con-tradiction in the effects of social class among and between different groups of the aged (e.g., the poor versus the affluent). On one hand, the importance of social class is both more visible and more significant for the aged living in an exclusive retirement community. The key concept here is "community." Rose says past sources of social status remain influential if the aged individual continues to live in the same community. There are, of course, many different kinds of communities. The affluent elderly have created a segregated upper-class social group where members are closely related economically, politi-cally, socially, and by kinship ties. It is a community of homogeneous "haves," where past sources of social status glow in the present and into the future.

On the other hand, a "community" of poor residents in inner city hotels subsidized by the United States Department of Housing and Urban Develop-ment (HUD) resides in a wide-open, unrestricted context in which tradition, heritage, lineage, manners, material wealth, and the genteel excuse of eccen-tricity are almost nonexistent. Residents of the HUD hotels have been forced to change communities—sometimes frequently—and for the old-timers in the area, the inner city has radically transformed around them. Past sources of social status are only hearsay. Thus a wildly heterogeneous collection of "have-nots" are obligated to downgrade the importance of former indicators of social status and re-evaluate or upgrade the worth of others, for example, physical health (Pelham 1980). Rose's hypothesis that physical and mental health may have special value in conferring status among the elderly—the existence of a subculture aside—finds a good deal of support in the HUD hotels.

Along this same line, Dowd (1980) offers some direction in understanding the effects of social class or statification per se; a few tentative observations on class, social inequality, power, dependency, and old age follow. First, growing old and poor clearly means a different quality of life compared to growing old affluently. The culture of class aside, *the aged rich are different because they have had more money throughout their entire lives.* Accumulated uneven distribution of a good physical aging is largely related to income or social class in its narrow sense. For a large number of the wealthy, there is a lifetime of good food, accessible, fine medical care, higher education, career paths linked to power, a positive self-image, and optimism. Nevertheless, we still know of affluent retirement communities that are truly gilt ghettoes in every sense of the word (FitzGerald 1983).

Second, the affluent aged can suffer just as much or more alcoholism, loneliness, waiting time, and powerlessness in exchange with *same class* age strata as their poor counterparts. This is an issue of social inequality.

Third, Dowd argues that power is linked to social structures, the interaction of people, and negotiated exchange rules based on resources. The net result is that "social class affects social exchange." Dowd's equation may have some validity when calling a cab to an affluent section of the city, but for the poor in the inner city, all the rules and contents of exchanges are rendered problematic. Individuals in the Tenderloin are not neatly linked to social structures; human interactions are not only a medium, but also a means to different ends, and the nature of the interaction is different; and valuable resources are not necessarily those traditionally valued in other contexts. Resources can be anything from a knife at your throat to an ability to talk your way gracefully out of a strong-arm robbery attempt.

Fourth, Dowd's conceptualization of dependence in social exchange correctly describes the relationship and power differential of apartment or hotel managers vis-à-vis apartment or hotel residents. Further, the concept of dependence can be generalized to include a state of being dependent upon institutional arrangements, for example, Supplemental Security Income. This is not to say that dependence is an individual trait or condition. It is a relative power differential between the aged individual and an individual or institution with more power resources.

Perhaps some of the muddle of stratification may be untangled by exploring the notion that age is an intervening variable, within and between age strata (e.g., age as a "leveler"). Anecdotal evidence suggests that in many contexts, downward mobility is associated with aging. Given this assumption, relative power and resources in an exchange relationship decline accordingly.

A particularly useful concept describing the power/dependency status of the aged was coined by Professor Leonard Schatzman (1982). "Kinstitution" is a dual concept of structural and interactional components. It represents a symbiotic cultural protection and caring for the aged and the notion of institution as Kin; that is, institutional arrangements providing all and/or supplementary support activities of families or friend networks.

Kinstitutions are curious hybrids in that they serve to foster dependence upon services and particular service structures, while at the same time providing needed care, respite for families, and independence from a forced-choice placement in a nursing home.

Schatzman's concept of kinstitution has also been employed elsewhere to describe the nature of community-based, long-term care agencies (Pelham and Clark 1986b).

Yet, even an enlightened attempt to keep frail elders independent and in their own homes in fact only substitutes one gatekeeper for another. Instead of being dependent upon one's daughter for daily meals, dressing, and bathing, the elder person is dependent upon a homemaker chore worker from an In-Home Supportive Services agency. The essential nature and power differential of the relationship remains essentially the same.

Although the economic picture has brightened for many of the aged in recent years (Schulz 1985), at retirement, income and power bases diminish. Large numbers of elder Americans are pushed by powerful socioeconomic forces onto lower rungs of the societal ladder. Many of the aged poor are still forced into institutional, urban, rural, psychological, and emotional ghettoes.

Subculture

In a third analytic framework, Rose (1965) takes the societal separation of the elderly argument one step further and suggests that increasingly the aged live within the context of a subculture. Unlike the theoretical concepts of role and stratification represented above, a subcultural framework breathes life into the interactions of social actors negotiating a social order in a social world.

Rose's analysis of the subculture of the aging argues that it "is a general one that cuts across other subcultures—those based on occupation, religion, sex, and possibly even ethnic identification . . . "

Rose's analytic framework operates at a relatively abstract societal level, but some parallels may be drawn between it and findings among the aged poor. First, in congregate living arrangements from nursing homes to board and care facilities to rent-subsidized apartments to retirement communities, there are large numbers of eligible elders with an opportunity for creating an aging subculture. This is particularly true for city senior's housing in the Housing and Urban Development hotels. Second, many of the poor aged are separated by a lack of options and opportunities. In the case of rent-subsidized senior housing, age segregation is an institutional creation. Third, in terms of ecomomic and social situations, most of the aged poor have a lot in common. This is not to say that the aged poor constitute a homogeneous lot—our vignettes illustrate their heterogeneity despite the leveling effects of age and economic status. What the aged poor have in common with each other are: economic dependency and whatever stigma that status attends in an individual's value system; limited and often shrinking resources that like-wise fix and diminish choices; smaller social worlds not shaped by indivdiual preferences; a perception that societal institutions, including social values, have been unkind toward the aged (a generalized negative out-group feeling); poorer health than their middle- and upper-class peers; and a lower quality of life because fewer alternatives.

Even given those opportunities for the creation of *aging subculture,* we have not observed its development. Even a sense of in-group "community" is the exception rather than the rule. This same pattern was specified in earlier research investigating dimensions of adaptation of Housing and Urban Development single-room occupants (SROs) done by Pelham (1980).

First, it did not appear that a general aging subculture, if it exists, cut across lines of social class. Elders living in the Tenderloin are by income and territorial definition relegated to the status of "lower class" and did not, as a rule, mix with their counterparts uptown. However, Rose is accurate in his point that where opportunity and conditions put old people of different social classes together, the class distinctions are likely to be less important. This was borne many times in the Tenderloin.

Although Rose recognizes the diminishing influence of wealth and pres-tige (if in fact it diminishes, and sometimes it does not) and the increasing value of mental and physical health, he does not "ground" the process within a specific social context. For example, losing a Social Security check and having diabetes in an uptown retirement community is qualitatively different from losing a Social Security check and having diabetes in a Tenderloin hotel. Also, elders in the HUD hotels did not necessarily experience an aging group consciousness based in part on a change in self-conception as progressively "physically and mentally handicapped," or moving from "independence to dependence" or "aspiring to declining." This is an empirical question and depends upon variations in adaptation and individual perception.

Finally, residents in HUD hotels had not developed a spontaneous, crys-tallized sense of belonging to an aging group. If anything, whatever exists had been largely imposed from outside by well-meaning youth and political interest groups like Gray Panthers. That is, although hotel residents were not observed to be particularly politically active in and of themselves, occasional visits by members of Gray Panthers highlighted current events and encouraged participation in partisan interest groups. Hotel residents know they are aged but do not think of themselves as "old" or "senior citizens." Such concepts suggest disability, or illness, or inadequacy. They realize they are relatively poor and share problems, but proudly think of themselves as *urban survivors*. In short, they behave politically like any other age group—according to perceived interests. If the issue is age-related—for example, lower bus fares for seniors, rent controls, or cutbacks in services—they formed groups for a time, applied pressure, and voted according to their own best interests. Organized, active, in-group elders may constitute a growing trend, but they remain a minority among the urban poor.

Even though hotel residents shared characteristics of age, values, public assistance, living arrangements, and residence in an island of safety in a hostile environment; they had *not* formed a subculture or community in the strictest sense. While elements of community were emerging, the HUD SROs remained an extremely heterogeneous lot.

Adaptation Frameworks

Various adaptation frameworks in gerontological literature attempt to specify successful aging. The work of Tobin and Lieberman (1976) examines adaptation to life crises in which an assessment of personal resources predicts adjustment to the stress of a change of residence. The adaptation to life crises model is multidimensional, accounting for environmental and interpersonal variables alike.

The only real area of conflict between this adaptive process framework and lives of the aged poor—and it is more a difference of quality than kind—rests in the relative weight placed upon degree of environmental change over personal resources, "coping skills," and perceptions of stress in predicting successful adaptation.

In terms of changing environment, the world of the old and poor can be near pandemonium—particularly in the inner city and transient hotels—yet amazing numbers of the aged not only adapt and survive but thrive there. On the surface, this suggests that personal resources are more important, particularly as they influence human interaction. The crucial question to be asked is not which external or internal variables are more significant, but *how are they perceived?* This process predicts their relative meaning and consequences.

A social labeling theory by Kuypers and Bengtson (1973) employs a social breakdown syndrome to explain and predict the relationship between individual maladaptation in old age and larger normative social structures.

This model is essentially identical to the deviance-as-labeling model except that an elder person has taken the place of the "offender" or "mentally ill" in the equation, or feedback loop in this case.

Numerous areas of disagreement exist between a labeling and social breakdown framework and observations of the old and poor. They tend to fall into the category of conflicting assumptions about the nature of humankind. Findings among the old and poor make clear that they are decidedly not "labeled" quivering masses of protoplasm absorbing negative external cues in order to form a self-concept. Role loss often means the creation of new roles; ambiguous normative guidance is not necessarily a negative condition and whether there is a lack of reference groups is an empirical question. There may in fact be powerful negative societal notions about growing old, but there is no evidence that these are either wholeheartedly internalized to be superimposed over pre-existing self-conceptions or instrumental in affecting a decline in competence.

Lieberman, Tobin, Kuypers, and Bengtson are all laboring under the common assumption that the aged are somehow fundamentally different from other human beings and human groups. It is presumed that the aged are victims, frail or weak, dependent and worse, and struggling in a hostile environment. These assumptions form implicit underpinnings to theory and subtly shape methodology and, in the end, conclusions.

Intentionality throughout human life cycle is the key concept in the adaptation model of Lowenthal, Thurnher, and Chiriboga (1975). The word "model" is used advisedly here as the study consists more of a collection of concepts than an explicit and fully specified model. Lowenthal and her associates essentially argue that individuals strive for intentionality—an adaptive process to make goals and behavior compatible—throughout the life course. It is further argued that "life stage" rather than age itself is a better predictor of stress and adaptation throughout the life cycle. It appears that intentionality is the dependent variable in this equation, but whether the dominant independent variable is stress or life stage is unclear. This is partly because the nature and number of stressors vary depending on the particular life stage.

Findings among the old and poor have no quarrel with the life stage model *per se*, but a word of caution is appropriate. While the old and poor indeed face challenges that are life-stage related, they would be hard pressed to fit themselves into four mutually exclusive categories of "presumed stress" and "numbers of negative feelings." Although the intentionality/life cycle model places an emphasis upon presumed stress, it still seems to somehow exist in a vacuum or hang in space without grounding. Where is the social context? It is, again, another example of a theoretical cookie cutter pressed against phenomena rather than the other way around.

The final adaptation model of House (1974) is probably the most integrated and comprehensive. It postulates five classes of variables: social conditions conducive to stress, perceived stress, response to stress (three kinds), outcomes (three kinds), and conditioning variables (three kinds). The model/paradigm is neat, testable, and intriguing. House's framework is in fact a medical model but it lends itself to a sociological application. It considers both structural and interactional categories.

A recent attempt at a modified House model has been undertaken by George (1980). Again, George's modified version has a structure stimulus/response orientation, but it makes the useful sociological reformulations of adding the concepts of identity adjustment, role, transitions, anomie, social status, and socialization.

Geoge's modified House model, and the original House version itself, share with the intentionality/life cycle model the problem of pre-existing categories above the ground. But, once again, where is social power?

The social adjustment in later life models go a long way toward better understanding the process of growing old, but they all seem to possess an inherent conservative bias: the theories are heavy with *a priori* assumptions; the reflexive nature of human group life is often lost in the analysis and the reality and implications of differential power is absent altogether.

Social Psychological Frameworks

One social psychological or developmental approach to the human life cycle (Neugarten 1968) has implications for adaptation in later life. Neugarten finds that human personality is essentially persistent and orderly throughout the life cycle; therefore patterns of aging are consistent with past modes of mastering the environment.

Our vignettes of the old and poor certainly support persistent personality patterns offered by Neugarten. Even if social worlds shrink or health fails, individuals continue behaviors and attitudes developed in the past and apply and adapt them to the present. This is particularly true for individuals living independently in the problematic environment of an inner city.

Many times city dwellers, as single room occupants, both explained and displayed that their personality and behavior patterns were consistent with earlier years. The seventy-year-old woman who breaks house rules by picking the lock on the back door and going out in her wheelchair was once a twenty-year-old woman who defied convention by going on stage as a dancer. Likewise, the timid thirty-year-old man who became a watchmaker against his will is the same eighty-year-old man who was forced to retire and who today cannot see the value of becoming involved with others and is simply waiting to die.

Our areas of disagreement with the psychology of the life-cycle approach concern the assumed nature of this "consistent personality" persona and the supposed differences between men and women. Our observations are that what the persona "looks like and does" is more like the past persona than unlike it. For example, there is no evidence of self-directed increase or heightened importance of introspection. Such a phenomenon may be a function of absent exterior stimuli (e.g., a job, young people to care for, or a role as a wise healer). With time on your hands in a small social space with few monetary or physical resources, what might you do?

Additionally, we found little evidence that most of the aged perceive the environment to be any more "complex" or "dangerous" than do thirty-year-olds. Whatever cautions or concerns exist, they are based upon empirical evidence and physical abilities and disabilities. If an individual is a homebody it is not necessarily because he wishes it to be so. Steep, rickety stairs, poor vision, and a lack of transportation are what make the environment complex or dangerous, not age per se.

Insofar as introspection and dangerous environment are concerned, consider this: a number of younger people are buying hand guns and putting up stocks of food in case of crime waves, earthquakes, or nuclear holocaust. Still others are searching for essential selves by way of hot tubs, vegetarianism, gurus, self-actualization therapy, divorce, sexual orientation experimentation, community living, meditation, vitamin therapy, drug use, running— or all of the above! Acting out introspective behaviors may be more common in California but it is certainly not age-specific.

Regarding Neugarten's psychology of the life cycle and differences between aged men and women, our study finds no indication or demonstration that poor men "cope with the environment in increasingly abstract and cognitive terms" or that women cope "in increasingly affective and expressive terms." This is not to say that personality changes do not occur throughout the life span; it only says that "coping," or adapting patterns, remain consistent and do not suddenly become sex-linked in old age.

Given sociocultural dimensions, individual personality, and personal biography, the aging experiences of women versus those of men are poorly understood. For every man who does not understand how to fill out a government form, there is a woman who is ignorant about preparing nutritionally sound meals. For every man who is afraid to venture out of the house there is a woman afraid to express her loneliness.

Yet this picture does not reflect the color of the lives of the vast majority of the old and poor. This impotent picture is an inaccurate depiction of elders who suffer the consequences of accumulated losses, but manage poverty, become streetwise, learn new roles (indeed, create them), and successfully adapt to the problems of chronic illness.

The keys to the differential responses in Rosow's sad world are: variations in adaptation and interpretations of reality.

As for the aging transition of women, the very existence of sharp role discontinuity in old age remains an empirical question—never mind whether it is more discontinuous for men or for women. Our findings suggest that social roles are evolving entities and selves are created or not created under certain conditions. Our observations indicate that roles *qua* roles do not always decline—for women or men. Women absolutely do not have the luxury of adapting to their roles (declining or otherwise) more slowly than men. The world of the old and poor is an unforgiving turf and women are faced with almost exactly the same structural and interpersonal dilemmas as men—controlling for gender-specific issues. It is impressive that women survive as well as they do.

Fontana (1977) has conducted an intriguing study in which the aged in various milieus were observed. Among these were the poor elderly.

Fontana's poor women and the women of our own study continue to defy a well-defined theory of aging. Significant numbers are disengaged in one way or another, but the status seems forced. At least equal numbers are active by magnifying everyday concerns, but this is not "leisure" in the sense of activity theory (i.e., self-directed leisure with options, not just passing time). Life cycle and developmental approaches can account for the pliable and lucky women who adapt, but miss the point with those who fall between the cracks not only in theory but also in reality.

The symbolic interactionist perspective of Fontana's seminal study has substantially influenced the wider field of gerontology. However, even interactionism lacks the emphasis on power relations in exchange theory.

Sociology of Knowledge Frameworks

The framework of the sociology of knowledge (Estes 1979) addresses issues surrounding the creation and consequences of social policy for the aged. It makes possible the bold leap that links abstract social policy and aging theory to grounded observations. This "grounding of theory" occurs in three greater to lesser abstract and analytically separate realms, which in reality are circular. They are:

1. Philosophical or domain assumptions about the nature of growing old
2. which form the underpinnings of theoretical assumptions about the aging process
3. which in turn shape ideologies, policies, and eventually everyday life.

(Everyday life then, of course, becomes the reality upon which the collective stock of knowledge about aging is based and the process has gone full circle).

In any case, in the first most abstract realm, findings in our study support the notion that the problems of growing old "are socially constructed as a result of our conceptions of aging and the aged" (Estes 1979).

In the second realm of inherent assumptions in gerontological theory, our observations among the poor suggest that the variable most absent in social theories of aging is power.

One theory of aging after another falls short in explaining the poor elderly and possesses a conservative bias because of the tendency to view individual experiences almost exclusively from the inside out. And, to be sure, the "inside" of the social actor in such a theory is most likely presumed to be weak, dependent, or ill—never mind how the individual got that way. We argue for a more balanced interactionist analysis. Such stereotypic generalizations and depictions of the aged find little corroboration in our study. It is a fallacy that the aged are somehow fundamentally different from other human beings and human groups. Again, in support of Estes, our research argues that "the inadequacy of much of the research on old age comes from its focus on what old people do rather than on the social conditions and policies that cause them to act as they do" (Estes 1979).

Marxist or Political Economy Analysis[1]

Certainly no theoretical consideration of aging would be complete without exploring issues related to a Marxist analysis.

From the Marxist point of view, the problem for aged in the United States and every industrialized nation is a relationship to the economic order. The secondary problem for the aged is the ideology that is both promoted by the industrial elite and emerges from political ecomomic structures and concomitant social structures and power relations.

Elements of this analysis argue that ideology, like knowledge, is socially generated and distributed. Intersubjective relation to the ideology depends upon geography, social class, education, employment, gender, religion, and more. Thus, during preindustrial epochs, the young and aged were more needed, albeit for labor. One might further argue that the young and aged were more loved and cared for because of what they were able to give in exchange. Power relations were more in balance, even given the ideology that human worth was linked to a very narrowly defined productivity.

For Marx, the sum total of productivity becomes the foundation upon which the cultural superstructure of society is built. Further, systems of production determine the nature of every element of society from fashion to religious faith. In short, social being determines consciousness.

So, today, the aged in all industrialized countries with a market economy find themselves with a problematic power differential. And as time goes on many elders find themselves sliding or pushed to the short end of the measuring stick of sociopolitical power.

We believe gerontology theorists would do well to consider the revelations of Kuhn (1970) and Gouldner (1970); that is, understand that *aging* is socially constructed; that *aging theory* and *theorists' minds* are socially constructed; and, that ideology is implicit in each and every analytic framework—including ours.

Further, we believe the chief problem of existing foregoing gerontological theory is that it is not self-conscious. Theorists are not aware that the nature of aging is shaped by their analytic kaleidoscopes.

For the most part, this discussion is a product of an exchange of ideas and analytic frameworks with Theodore Keller, Ph.D., professor of political science at San Francisco State University. Dr. Keller is an international scholar, author, and teacher and has recently turned his analytic skills to the area of aging.

12
Planning and Policies

General Observations

What do the foregoing chapters and vignettes teach us about the nature of poverty among the aged in the United States? What directions do they point to for planners and creators of social policy?

First, we did not find a so-called "tangle of pathology" among the old and poor and their families. We found examples of individuals from all walks of life who simply outlived their limited resources or found their resources inadequate in an inflationary market economy.

Second, elders living in poverty tended to suffer a higher incidence of health problems—but such is the case with low-income people of all ages. While these elder survivors have had time to both develop and adapt to poor health, we cannot help but wonder about the fate of those who did not. Looking back, chronic illness may be the only legacy left for the poor elder.

Third, the personal histories confirm that personality remains relatively constant. Patterns of interaction with self, others, and social forces—both large and small—are persistent over a lifetime. There is no "tangle of pathology" in the areas of mental health and competence either.

Fourth, many of our poor elders spent a lifetime teetering on the edge of poverty. They always existed on the margin, "one paycheck away from poverty." Many of the old and poor were earlier the young and poor, and the young and near-poor. Later, when they did receive that last paycheck or their spouses died, they slipped into the maw of poverty.

An Aside

When our team was discussing the repeating scenario of "slipping" into poverty, we raised the question of the social construction of both the concept of poverty and acquiring the status. A critical look at the language employed to describe this status passage is enlightening. So many of the verbs describe the status passage as something that occurs relatively suddenly—like a trap door dropping open, (slipped, fell, sank into poverty). The individual actor is described alternatively as a helpless victim or pathological creature who somehow deserves the fate.

Our observations of the old and poor are that the elder individual living in poverty is neither a helpless victim nor pathological creature. She (and it is usually a woman) is most likely an able citizen who struggled a lifetime against institutional arrangements stacked against her. She did not slip into poverty; she was dragged kicking, scratching, and screaming. From the woman's point of view, she was pushed into poverty by powerful social forces like lack of fertility control, insufficient and low-pay employment without maternity leave, little or no child care, limited educational opportunites, poor health care, and absent retirement plans.

Yet, even given the heroic struggles of elders against the odds in these vignettes, the old and poor lie psychologically within normal ranges. Each individual here will fit under the proverbial bell curve.

Interventions

After reviewing the old and poor, we find the problem is quite simply a lack of money. Therefore, the solution is quite simply increasing income. We recommend intervention at very early ages. For example, the quintessence of a future lifetime of poverty is a pregnant, single, ethnic minority high school drop-out.

Historically, the policy instrument has been services. We wish to ask, why not money?

Social Security is a pay-as-you-go system. Entitlement programs are, for the most part, designed to support status quo institutional arrangements and existing power relations among social groups—the so-called "infamy of the status quo." Social service and health care dollars flow into the hands of providers, not elders themselves. If there is a "tangle of pathology," it exists among some services providers who are maximizing self-interests.

Raising incomes of elders will allow them to be autonomous units, advocates for independence. Elders can purchase needed services when, where, for what, and from whom they choose. The literature clearly supports the idea most older adults—even the frail—can manage their affairs with competence. Further, when an elder needs support, usually an involved, responsible informal support system responds. (We would do well to address our research and concern toward the overworked and overlooked informal support providers.)

Arguments that the elderly somehow differ from the rest of us, that they need protection from themselves (except in very special limited circumstances), are flawed. This reasoning rests on the myth that elders are incompetent.

Public Policy: Promote the General Welfare

Ideology about the nature of aging produces national programs directed at the aged. Critical scrutiny of ideology finds it contains myths, assumptions, sacred and profane doctrine, values and more. Sociologically speaking, ideology is a set of beliefs that legitimize social stratification and social structures. Idology is so deeply ingrained in our consciousness that it rarely rises to a level of questioning. Ideology is reflexive and circular in the sense it is both a product of and produces consciousness.

Interest groups socially construct ideology in human groups. Like knowledge, it is socially distributed. Ideologies exist in a status hierarchy, with the dominant ideology created by the powerful and usually justifying economic interests. As a simple but compelling example, ideologies have historically provided legitimacy to all manner of behaviors and public laws that discriminated against certain classes of U.S. citizens. Today's racism, sexism, and ageism illustrate the human and social costs of ideologies that appeared part of the natural order in their day.

Ageism is perhaps the newest member of the "ism" family. A critical examination of ageism as created by a dominant ideology poses some interesting questions. Racism, sexism, and ageism represent belief systems that legitimize social inequality based upon biological characteristics. Once we have that notion clearly in mind as an analytic framework, the nature of social policy in the United States becomes clear.

Income

Income programs for the aged in the United States consist of Social Security, other retirement plans (e.g., military and federal civilian), and Supplemental Security Income. States have an optional "add-on" called State Supplemental Payment.

Social Security is not what its name implies. Social Security does not provide sufficient income to protect the aged from destitution in later years.

The original intent of Social Security was to insure adequate income for older Americans. Social Security was meant to remedy a societal phenomenon of scandalous poverty suffered by older Americans who had left the workforce. (Recall that public and private retirement plans were relatively new.) Without incomes, and because goods and services must be purchased in the United States, older Americans were relegated to damnation.

Social Security itself was the direct result of ideology and interest group politics. One of the stated values of the United States is to promote the general welfare.

However, the "solution" of Social Security was an outgrowth of work ethic and political economy ideologies. Enacted in 1935 during Franklin D. Roosevelt's first term, the Social Security Act was the result of political compromises. Some groups wanted universal coverage and liberal benefits while other groups wanted to severely limit any federal involvement in such a social insurance plan. A system whereby older citizens would ascribe to a sacred status to be given societies' treasures did not emerge. Rather, older Americans were required to earn Social Security by labor and in turn buy the necessities of life. Food, clothing, and shelter had to be purchased.

The existence of Supplemental Security Income provides evidence of the inadequacies and gaps in Social Security. SSI is designed to provide a national minimum federal payment to the aged and disabled and is directed at the low-income aged.

Structurally, this two-class arrangement for income separates out non-workers, under-employed, and disabled individuals who receive SSI. They are by definition segregated. Here, low-income elders are by statute relegated to "other-classness," if not "lower-classness".

Our aged interviewees in the vignettes expressed a perceived "outsider/stranger" status. Even given the meager income provided by SSI/SSP and cost-of-living adjustments, our elders found themselves without enough money. Elders were forced to supplement their income with odd jobs like Judy Anderson's doll making or employ painful money-conserving devices like Agnes Hughes and Albert Shaw.

Health Care

The two-class pattern repeats in the health care structures of Medicare and Medicaid. Looking at Medicare and Medicaid through the analytic framework of ideology, we see the charge to protect the health of the aged takes the form of an umbilicus that provides a direct flow of public dollars to social structures (Part A Hospital and Part B Physician) created by a dominant medical ideology. Medicare stipulates that health care be provided by physicians in hospitals with an emphasis on technology-dependent acute care. This biased argument exists in contrast to the weight of evidence that chronic and long-term care are the most frequent and pressing health care concerns of the aged (even without considering issues of prevention and health promotion, which are even further removed from acute care).

With the advent of Medicaid for the low income, health care has evolved into a four-tier system: private pay with or without Medicare and "medi-gap" insurance; Medicare with or without "medi-gap" insurance; Medicaid; and the uninsured. The National Council on the Aging reports that 40 million divorced, retired, or widowed individuals face catastrophe should they become seriously ill before reaching the age for Medicare coverage.

Medicaid differs from Medicare in that it provides for long-term care. However, the prejudice for institutional settings prevails. In fact, the nursing home industry itself originated from the same umbilicus of public dollars. But in the case of Medicaid, still another industry blossomed, consisting of armies of "gatekeepers," managers, and costcutters.

Today, "cost-sharing," the Prospective Payment System, and a Medicaid "cap" are examples of ideologies colliding after the creation of a Frankenstein medical monster. Industries have grown gigantic—even bloated—by the umbilicus of public dollars. Policy makers and interest groups promoting cost containment now search for ways to reduce costs.

As we follow the trail of ideology as predictor of possible futures, we find that cost controls are now primarily aimed at elder recipients and that responsibility is shifting to the community. Medical institutional arrangements are essentially left intact.

Rendering the whole configuration problematic, a purist might suggest an umbilicus that provides a direct flow of public dollars into the hands of elders who may choose the nature and setting of health care.

Present Expenditure Patterns

Much has been made of the federal government's relatively large expenditures for the elderly. For federal fiscal year 1986, the current estimate is about $290 billion (U.S. Congress 1986). The distribution of these expenditures, by programmatic component, is shown in figure 12–1.

The income transfers, a total of $190.5 billion, are mostly made up of Social Security payments ($144.5 billion) and other retirement programs (e.g., the military). Also included is the $4.1 billion that the Supplemental Security Income program provides the elderly and disabled.

The health care component of $86.6 billion is largely composed of Medicare ($74.5 billion), Parts A and B, portions of the Veterans Administration's medical programs, and a portion of the Medicaid program used by the elderly.

These two components, income and health, make up 96 percent of all outlays to the elderly.

Housing makes up 2 percent; medical research (e.g., the National Institute on Aging) another 1 percent; and services the last 1 percent.

Single purpose taxes (i.e., Social Security withholding tax) finance 84 percent of these outlays, about $2.4 billion (figure 12–2). In other words,

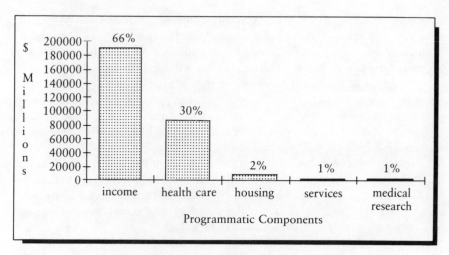

Figure 12–1. Two-thirds of federal outlays for the elderly are income transfers, federal fiscal year 1986

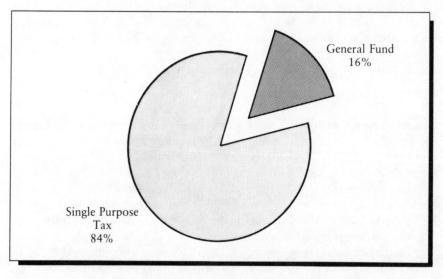

Figure 12–2. 84 percent of federal outlays for the elderly are financed through single purpose taxes, federal fiscal year 1986

almost all programs for the elderly are self-financed and are not dependent on general revenue taxes. This means these expenditures are outside the bookkeeping that accounts for the federal deficit. Because these monies are kept in trust accounts and cannot be used for any other purposes, policy makers looking for ways to reduce the federal deficit should not look toward

Social Security or Medicare. *These programs did not contribute to the deficit in the first place and simply are not part of the deficit-making process.*

Figure 12–2 shows single purpose taxes such as Social Security and Medicare Hospital Insurance finance almost all outlays and very little is financed through general tax revenues. Medical care programs (e.g., the elderly's share of Medicaid) take up two-thirds of the general-tax-financed programs.

Specific Recommendations for Change

Two major characteristics differentiate the elderly poor from their more affluent peers: less income and poorer physical health. Otherwise, we found the old and poor to be actively engaged with their families and friends and within the ranges of "normal" psychological well-being. Our recommendations focus on three areas: income transfer, medical care coverage, and nonmedical services.

Each year since 1972, over 3 million elderly consistently fall below the official Census Bureau definition of poverty. This situation continues to exist despite the declining rate of poverty among the elderly. As figure 12–3 data show, since 1972, the poverty rate declined from 18.6 percent to 12.4 per-

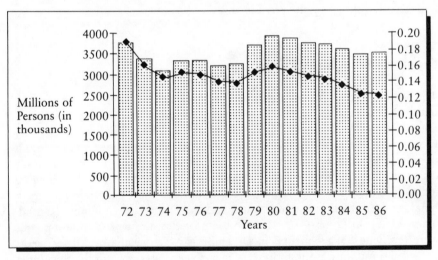

Sources: U.S. Bureau of the Census. Money income and poverty status of families and persons in the United States: 19*nn*.. Current Population Survey. P-60, Nos. 116, 127, 134, 140, 145, 149, 154, and 157. Washington, D.C.: U.S. Government Printing Office.

Figure 12–3. Number of 65 + population below poverty line, 1972–1986, and declining poverty rate, U.S.

cent in 1986, but the total number of impoverished elderly remained between 3 and 4 million people—varying from 3.9 million in 1980 to 3.1 million in 1974.

This fourteen-year-old pattern implies that a hard-core permanently poor aged group exists in the United States, only marginally sensitive to what happens at the macro level of the economy or what public policies are implemented. Although some movement may occur in and out of poverty by a few elderly, this movement is likely to be a statistical artifact and the "escape" not permanent (Holden, et al. 1986), because the usual means of escaping poverty—a job, higher wages, or marriage—are not readily available to the aged poor. Once they become "officially" poor, it usually means poor, or near-poor, for the rest of their lives. If a person reaches age sixty-five and is poor, then this means a "lifetime" of about another fifteen to twenty years. As they age, they will even become more poor, the highest poverty rates are among the "old-old."

The major economic and demographic structural causes of impoverishment are well-known—patterns of occupational segregation and discriminatory compensation schedules (Pearce 1978) and widowhood (Morgan 1986; Zick and Smith 1986)—and we will not dwell on them here. Our present purposes are to review the major public policy instrument aimed at assisting low-income elderly—the Supplemental Security Income program—and to propose a means of eliminating poverty among the 3 to 4 million elderly who consistently fall below the poverty threshold.

Supplemental Security Income Program

The Social Security Amendments of 1972 (Public Law 92-603) established a national program with uniform payment standards and eligibility requirements for the needy aged, blind, and disabled. The Supplemental Security Income program replaced the federally assisted, state-administered programs of old-age assistance, aid to the blind, and aid to the permanently and totally disabled. The primary objective of the program was to provide, through a federally administered program, a minimum income to the nation's aged, blind, and disabled in the fifty states and the District of Columbia (Grundmann 1985). In January 1974, when the program began, 3.2 million people were receiving SSI payments. In December 1985, the number of recipients exceeded 4 million; 1.5 million were in the aged category and the remainder were in the blind and disabled categories. Of the blind and disabled, an additional 586,783 were over age sixty-four (25,489 blind and 561,294 disabled) (Kahn 1987).

State supplementation payments may be either mandatory or optional. Mandatory state supplementation refers to payments required to maintain the income level of recipients who were transferred from the former state programs to SSI. Optional supplementary payments are provided to augment payment levels of all or selected categories of recipients. Optional state supplementation plans vary widely. As of December 1985, one in four of the aged recipients had been converted from a previous state-administered program (Kahn 1987).

As the country's major income-maintenance policy for the poor elderly financed from general revenue sources, SSI has three major flaws. The first is an extremely low participation rate among the aged poor—well below 50 percent of those eligible receive benefits. The second is a set of administrative rules that unduly restrict eligibility. The third is an inadequate benefit level.

Participation Rate

No consensus prevails about the exact level of participation of the poor aged in the SSI program. No official estimates are available from the Social Security Administration even though it publishes an annual report on the social and demographic characteristics of the SSI recipients. Researchers have to rely on secondary sources and samples to calculate the rate. These indirect methods invariable produce different estimates. For example, when we examine Census Bureau tables, we estimate the participation rate to be 23 percent among the aged poor (U.S. Bureau of the Census, table 11, 1985a). Louis Harris and Associates (1986) estimate that 17 percent of the elderly below the poverty line actually report receiving SSI. A recent Villers Foundation report (1987), citing U.S. Census data, states that among elderly households—not individuals—only 32 percent participate in the SSI program. The Commonwealth Fund Commission on Elderly People Living Alone (1987), based on numbers provided by ICF, Inc., estimates program participation to be 34 percent.

Possible explanations for the low rate of participation include lack of information about the program and its benefit structure; an individual's health and financial status; avoidance of the welfare bureaucracy and the stigma of receiving public assistance; and low benefits. Whatever the reasons and whatever the "true" rate of participation, it is certainly low. We can safely say that fewer than half of the poor elderly receive SSI payments. In fact, it appears that the rate has dropped from higher levels of about 50 percent (Coe 1985) to its present lower rate. As a chief component of the welfare "safety net," the SSI program fails to "catch" more than half of its potential population. The "porosity" of the safety net has been examined and noted elsewhere (Uehara et al. 1986).

Finally, as can be expected with a declining participation rate, the SSI caseload for the aged has also declined steadily since its initial phase-in period, 1974–75. By 1980, the caseload had dropped below the number of recipients being paid old-age assistance in 1973 prior to the first SSI payments. The present 1987 caseload level falls below the pre-SSI levels as well. The caseload decline is commonly attributed to mortality, increased Social Security benefits, increased number of elders sixty-five or older counted as disabled and blind beneficiaries, and less intensive outreach efforts (Menefee et al. 1981).

Rules

The second major flaw with the SSI program has to do with eligibility rules, the most important of which states that an individual can only have countable assets of eighteen hundred dollars and, for a couple, twenty-seven hundred dollars (as of 1987). The original ceilings, fixed in 1972, were fifteen hundred dollars and two thousand dollars. Even though the ceilings are scheduled to increase to two thousand dollars for an individual and three thousand dollars for a couple by January 1989, they have not kept up with inflation. Potential program participants are excluded because SSI didn't index for inflation. This exclusionary power can best be illustrated by the low participation rate among the poor as determined by the U.S. Census, 23 percent, since the census only counts cash income and not assets.

Another rule reduces benefits by one-third if the SSI recipient lives in the household of another for a full month and receives maintenance and support. The net effect of the reduction may mean to the potential recipient that it is not worth the administrative hassle—the "transaction costs"—to continue with the program or to make initial contact with a possibly intrusive welfare bureaucracy.

Benefit Level

Those poor aged who do receive SSI have found that its maximum benefit levels fall below the poverty level. For example, for 1987, the maximum federal SSI benefit for an individual was 76 percent of the poverty threshold; for a couple, the benefit represented 90 percent of the threshold (Commonwealth Fund Commission 1987). As of January 1986, only 20 percent of the aged individuals and 24 percent of couples received the maximum monthly SSI payment (Kahn 1987). Even with the state supplementary payments, only four states—Alaska, California, Connecticut, and Massachusetts—have maximum benefit levels that raise individuals above the poverty threshold. Thirteen states have programs that raise a couple above the threshold. The simple explanation is that SSI was not designed to eliminate poverty—just to provide a national minimum income.

A Simple Proposal

Our proposal to eliminate poverty among the aged is simply to give them enough cash to reach the poverty threshold. For reasons we indicated earlier, the SSI program, as presently structured, is not the policy instrument of choice. Besides reaching fewer than half the aged poor, a recent study (Zedlewski and Meyer 1987) estimated that even if the SSI benefit level were raised to the poverty threshold, the simulated response would only increase program participation by 3 percent (Commonwealth Fund Commission 1987). This 3 percent increase would be the long-run effect, representing the best estimate about future participation behavior. The short-run effect is actually estimated to be a decrease in program participation—from 48 percent to 45 percent—because the pool of program eligibles increases immediately while the behavioral response lags. The study does not provide any specific time periods for short-run and long-run effects.

Although the poverty rate for the aged would drop to about 8 percent, over 2 million aged would still be poor even if the SSI benefit level were raised to the poverty threshold. In the long run, 1 million to 2 million elderly would still be poor. Clearly, the SSI program, as presently structured, cannot solve the problem of poverty among the elderly by raising the benefit level to the poverty threshold.

Specifically, we propose to modify the SSI program with a "Gero-assistance Program" (GAP) payment to be made to all those aged sixty-five and older who receive Social Security benefits below the poverty threshold by an amount that would raise them to the poverty threshold. SSI, as it affects the nonaged blind and disabled, would remain the same.

An example of how the GAP payment would work is as follows. The average individual benefit check for all widows, poor and nonpoor, through the old-age, survivors, and disability insurance (OASDI) program, was $430.62 in December 1985 (Social Security Bulletin 1986). The poverty level for the aged individual in 1985 was $437.92. This individual would receive a separate GAP payment of $7.30, or an annual total of $87.60. For the 82.9 percent of the aged poor individuals already receiving OASDI checks (U.S. Congress 1986a), the GAP payment would raise them to at least the poverty threshold.

Within one month of implementation of the GAP payments, the poverty rate among the aged would drop to approximately 2 percent from its present level of about 13 percent.

For those 17.1 percent of the aged poor who do not receive Social Security benefits, SSI benefit levels would also be raised to the poverty level. (There exists some evidence that a large portion of this 17.1 percent is already enrolled in SSI, since one of the major explanatory variables of SSI participation is need. Those without any OASDI benefits are probably those most in need.)

GAP would not be means-tested; rather, it would be an entitlement without any assets ceilings. A few lines of computer program code—identifying the individuals and generating the GAP checks—would perform the eligibility determination function. The current corps of eligibility workers could be redirected to find and enroll the 17.1 percent of the aged poor not linked to OASDI.

No doubt, GAP payments would go to some individuals with high levels of financial resources. But, in these cases, the GAP payment would be treated as 100 percent taxable income after some threshold level of personal income. It is plausible that these individuals would view the checks as nuisances and order them stopped. Over time, this coverage would be self-correcting to a degree. The gain in administrative efficiency caused by reliance on computer-generated amounts and checks far outweighs the costs of the human effort (with sometimes dehumanizing results) it would take to prevent these exceptions.

Our GAP proposal may seem similar to the "double-decker" plan considered by the 1979 National Advisory Council on Social Security but it is significantly different. The differences are that the GAP payment replaces the current SSI payment and is explicitly tied to the poverty level. It is not a minimum Social Security payment. GAP is an administratively minimalist proposal that does not involve itself in the inner workings of Social Security benefit calculations; GAP does not affect the regular OASDI benefit amount and, under this proposal, the principal of "what you got is what you get," would rule so no one would be adversely affected; and GAP costs considerably less than the double-decker proposal, estimated to be $50 billion in 1979 (U.S. Congress 1980).

Costs

The price tag to eliminate poverty among the aged is $7 billion a year (1986 dollars). To arrive at this figure, we examined the latest available published U.S. Census data that calculates the average income deficit between actual income and the poverty threshold, the so-called "poverty gap." For 1984, the average (mean) for an unrelated individual, rather than a family, was $2,274—about $190 a month (U.S. Census, table 26, 1985a). (We used the mean rather than the median, a lesser amount of $1,750, because we do not know if the income deficit data clusters at the center of the distribution. If it did, then the median would not be as reliable as the mean. If we had used the median, the final answer would have been $4.3 billion instead of $6.6 billion [1984 dollars]).

During 1984, more than 2.4 million unrelated aged persons lived under the poverty threshold (U.S. Census, table 11, 1985a). The total annual cost for unrelated individuals, then, is $5.6 billion.

Similarly, for couples, in those families without children younger than eighteen years old (our proxy for the aged couple since the Census "poverty gap" data is not age-adjusted), the per-family-member income deficit was $1,182—about $99 a month. There were 855,000 aged persons who were married and below the poverty threshold in 1984; their total annual cost is $1 billion. The total new cost of the two groups then becomes $6.6 billion. This cost is in addition to the already existing level of federal SSI payments to the aged, approximately $4.2 billion, and $1.1 billion to the aged from the state supplemental programs. The grand total, then, for eliminating poverty among the aged is $11.9 billion—$6.6 billion in new funds and $5.3 billion in existing support levels.

This base calculation was done in 1984 dollars to facilitate replication and corroboration. Correcting for inflation according to the CPI (3.5 percent in 1985 and 3.2 percent in 1986), the amounts in 1986 dollars are a grand total of $12.7, with $7 billion as new monies.

Administration

The Social Security Administration would administer GAP. Because over 80 percent of the checks would be generated automatically by the SSA's computers, the existing eligibility work force would focus on those eligible persons not linked to OASDI. They would also focus on problem-solving efforts related to those aged individuals receiving blind or disabled benefits, but whose GAP payments may be more or less than they currently receive through SSI. Obviously a "hold-harmless" provision for these persons would have to be stipulated so as not to create inequities.

The actual GAP payment check would be separate from the Social Security check. The accounting and bookkeeping systems of the two programs would be separate. This would insure accountability of the program and would not endanger the actuarial soundness of the OASDI trust accounts by commingling and transferring between accounts. The only connection between GAP and OASDI would be the electronic linkage necessary to identify GAP recipients and to calculate check amounts. This could be done on a tape-to-tape basis or by other technologically appropriate means. The internal integrity of the OASDI computer systems would not be compromised.

Financing

The additional federal share created by GAP would represent about a 3 percent increase to the level of expenditures of general revenue-financed programs. We believe this is an acceptable price to pay for the elimination of poverty among the aged. Revenues for GAP payments could be generated by reducing national defense, cutting discretionary outlays for agricultural or business subsidies, or adopting any of the financing options described in the cited Zedlewski and Meyer report, such as restoring the estate tax thresholds to 1985 levels or changing the tax treatment of Social Security benefits.

Because several of the structural causes of poverty among the aged stem from local practices (e.g., discriminatory hiring and firing policies and compensation schedules), we believe GAP payments should be financed through a fifty-fifty sharing with the states to more equitably shoulder the cost. No increase would be needed for those four states with supplemental programs that already raise the individual above the poverty threshold, or for those thirteen states that already raise couples above the line. All states, when considering the total amount from the federal SSI benefit and the state supplement for the aged, fall within 75 percent of the poverty threshold for individuals and all are within 90 percent of the poverty threshold for couples (Commonwealth Fund Commission 1987). The increase necessary to bring them to 100 percent of the level would not represent a significant augmentation.

Interaction with Other Means-tested Programs

One of the major programs that interacts with SSI is Medicaid, the state-administered health insurance program for low-income people of all ages. In general, when one becomes eligible for SSI one is Medicaid eligible. However, Medicaid is a state-administered program and some states stipulate restrictive eligibility criteria, creating a confusing array of categorical groups and income levels, excluding many poor people of all ages (Brown 1984). The U.S. Census estimates (1987a) only 39.8 percent of the aged poor participate in Medicaid. As we have seen, the SSI program participation among the aged poor is low. By extension, this low rate affects the Medicaid program participation rate.

However, recent federal legislation (the Omnibus Budget Reconciliation Act of 1986, H. R. 5300) permits states to offer Medicaid coverage to all elderly and disabled up to a state-established poverty level that does not exceed 100 percent of the federal poverty level. If those states that created the "confusing array" of eligibility standards adopt this simpler criterion, then the interaction effect with GAP would be moot.

No doubt some states would want to retain Medicaid eligibility structures and processes to limit expenditures in that open-ended program. However, participation in Medicaid should be based on pre-GAP income levels. The recipient's Medicaid status should not be compromised.

This "hold-harmless" approach also should be used with other means-tested programs (e.g., food stamps). We do not propose to finance GAP payments through "offsets" from other service programs for the low-income elderly.

Limitations

The GAP proposal has several limitations we wish to acknowledge. First, it only deals with a small portion—the elderly—of the impoverished in the United States and does not deal with blind and disabled SSI recipients who are younger than sixty-five. Second, by following the official Census Bureau definition of poverty for the elderly, it perpetuates the two-level definition that discriminates against the elderly (Schulz 1985). Third, it does not address the needs of the near-poor—those individuals who are within 125 percent and 150 percent of the poverty threshold. Fourth, it does not deal with the structural processes that produce poverty in the first place. Although our approach runs counter to the dominant ideologies described earlier because of its cash rather than services nature, it does not deal directly with these ideologies. As such, it could be viewed as a palliative and as a distraction from the basic problems in the United States' socioeconomic structures.

There is no "however" to these limitations. They are real and we do not address them because our purpose here is to present a proposal and outline the means by which it can be implemented to achieve our immediate goal—the elimination of poverty among American's aged. Short-term and long-term solutions are not necessarily mutually exclusive. Finally, we emphatically state that the elimination of poverty, in an "official" statistical sense, still means that millions of elderly will continue to live in impoverished circumstances and will continue to need federal and state assistance, particularly in housing and medical care.

Medical Care Coverage

The second recommendation follows from the first. If poverty no longer exists among the elderly then we no longer need a separate medical insurance program for the poor elderly. We can eliminate Medicaid for the elderly and add those services which were covered by Medicaid to those covered by Medicare. The two most important Medicaid services used by the elderly are nursing home care and prescription drugs. The Harvard Medicare Project (1986) recently made a similar proposal but did not call for the abolition of Medicaid for the elderly. However, we see no need to retain it, given poverty would no longer exist among the elderly. Eliminating Medicaid for the elderly would not only do away with the two-tier medical care system but also would simplify the paperwork at the individual level and at the macro level. Without the elderly's participation in the Medicaid program—they account for about 37 percent of expenditures—the program could better focus on its prime users: mothers and children. The Medicaid program would become more of a maternal and child health program for the low income. With this emphasis, perhaps more progress could be made in reducing the high black infant mortality rates.

Financing the inclusion of these two major services—nursing home care and prescription drugs—would be accomplished by shifting the general revenues that had gone to Medicaid for them and making those funds available to Medicare; by increasing the payroll tax deduction to finance a new Part of Medicare—Part C, Long-term Care; and by beneficiary copayments. Exact proportions for each of these three mechanisms would no doubt be worked out in Congressional bargaining sessions. Suffice to say the total price tag would be an additional $10 to $20 billion by the year 2000. This is not a trivial amount. Legislators may have to "bite the political bullet" and vote for some kind of higher payroll tax deduction if we care to provide adequate and equitable medical care to the elderly. Similar political behavior occurred with recent reforms to Social Security. It can happen.

Two final notes about this proposal. First, with Medicare coverage of nursing home care, a danger of overuse exists because of government financing. Although others suggest a system of "gatekeepers" to control appropriate access to nursing home care, we do not advocate the creation of more "gerocrats" who would bureaucratically administer these channels. We know the nursing home placement decision is a "last resort" taken by families and is not likely to be abused by them. A more efficient way to control use is to limit the supply side. Emphasis should be placed on the certificate of need process so that the number of available nursing home beds will be closely monitored and expansion controlled to some degree.

Lastly, this proposal assumes that the basic delivery system of medical care in the United States remains essentially intact. Previous reforms of the whole medical care complex have indicated that it is "like squeezing a half-filled balloon—if you put pressure one place, it will get bigger somewhere else." If incremental reforms, such as those we have suggested and as others have suggested, do not bring about the desired effects, then serious consideration should be given to a form of national health insurance program, removing forever the present fee-for-service bias. Major ideological battles will result if support for a national health insurance program, such as one we outline elsewhere (Pelham and Clark 1986c), comes about. These battles will no doubt take us into the next century.

Services

As we saw in chapter 6, our respondents fall into two distinct groups: those who use services and those who do not. About two-thirds of our respondents did not use one nonmedical service and a similar pattern existed in the area of medical services. Also, almost one-half did not experience a transition between residency settings. These patterns tell us two distinct groups exist among the old and poor. One group, the minority, uses services while the other does not. It is an open question whether this second group *needs* services.

These use patterns suggest the term "continuum of care" may be misleading since it implies an orderly sequence of events and an equal distribution of resources along the continuum. Our analyses show that the actual experience of the elderly is more "off and on," more of a bi-modal distribution, and that the "users" of the services are clustered among a relatively small group. The implication for planners and policy makers may be to reformulate the array of services to focus in on "transition points" (e.g., home to hospital and hospital to home) to better target existing resources and to more efficiently assist those in need.

References

Aaron, H. J. 1978. *Politics and the Professors: The Great Society in Perspective.* Washington, D.C.: Brookings Institution.

Adams, D. L. 1969. "Analysis of a Life Satisfaction Index." *Journal of Gerontology* 24:470–474.

Allison, P. D. 1984. *Event History Analysis: Regression for Longitudinal Event Data.* Sage University Paper series on Quantitative Applications in the Social Sciences, 07–046. Beverly Hills and London: Sage Publications.

American Association of Retired Persons. 1985. *A Profile of Older Americans: 1985.* Washington, D.C.: American Association of Retired Persons.

Antonucci, T. C. 1985. "Personal Characteristics, Social Support, and Social Behavior." *In,* E. Shanas and R. H. Binstock (eds), *Handbook of Aging and the Social Sciences* (2nd ed.), New York, N.Y.: Van Nostrand.

Applebaum, D. K. 1977. "The Level of the Poverty Line: A Historical Survey." *Social Service Review* 51:514–523.

Ball, D. W. 1972. "The Family as a Sociological Problem: Conceptualization of the Taken-For-Granted as Prologue to Social Analysis." *Social Problems* 19:295–307.

Bengtson, V. L. 1979. "Ethnicity and Aging: Problems and Issues in Current Social Science Inquiry." *In* D. E. Gelfand and A. J. Kutzik (eds.) *Ethnicity and Aging.* New York, N.Y.: Springer Publishing Co.

Berger, P. L. and Luckman, T. 1966. *The Social Construction of Reality.* Garden City, N.Y.: Doubleday.

Bloom, M. 1975. "Evaluation Instruments: Tests and Measurements in Long Term Care." *In* S. Sherwood (ed.) *Long Term Care: A Handbook for Researchers, Planners, and Providers.* New York, N.Y.: Spectrum Publication.

Brown, E. R. 1984. "Medicare and Medicaid: The Process, Value, and Limits of Health Care." *In* M. Minkler and C. L. Estes (eds.) *Readings in the Political Economy of Aging.* Farmingdale, N.Y.: Baywood Publishing Co., Inc.

Burke, V. J., and V. Burke. 1974. *Nixon's Good Deed: Welfare Reform.* New York, N.Y.: Columbia University Press.

Butler, L. H., and P. W. Newacheck. 1981. "Health and Social Factors Relevant to Long-Term-Care Policy." *In,* J. Meltzer, F. Farrow, and H. Richman (eds.) *Policy Options in Long-Term Care.* Chicago, Ill.: The University of Chicago Press.

California. 1983. "The Feminization of Poverty: Facts and Figures." Sacramento, Calif.: Commission on the Status of Women.

———. 1984. *In-home Supportive Services, March 1983 Survey, Selected Characteristics.* Program Information Series Report No. 1984-07, Sacramento, Calif.: Department of Social Services.

———. 1985. "Long-Term Care in California." Sacramento, Calif.: Department of Health Services.

Cantor, M. H. 1979. "Neighbors and Friends." *Research on Aging* 1: 434–463.

Chiang, C. L. 1980. *An Introduction to Stochastic Processes and Their Applications.* Huntington, N.Y.: Robert E. Krieger Publishing Co.

Clark, M. L., L. Walter, and L. S. Miller. 1983. "Estimates of Medical Services Cost: Medi-Cal and Medicare Paid Claims—1981." Berkeley: MSSP Evaluation, University Extension, University of California, Berkeley, mimeo.

Clark, M. L., L. Walter, and L. S. Miller. 1982. "Medi-Cal Payments in MSSP, Phase I: A Preliminary Analysis," Berkeley: MSSP Evaluation, University of California Extension, mimeo.

Coe, R. D. 1985. "Nonparticipation in the SSI Program by the Eligible Elderly." *Southern Economic Journal* 3: 891–897.

Committee on an Aging Society. 1985. *Health in an Older Society.* Washington, D.C.: National Academy Press.

Commonwealth Fund Commission on Elderly People Living Alone. 1987. *Old, Alone and Poor.* Baltimore, Md.: The Commonwealth Fund Commission on Elderly People Living Alone.

Cumming, E., and W. Henry. 1961. *Growing Old.* New York, N.Y.: Basic Books.

Dasen, P. R. (ed). 1977. *Piagetian Psychology: Cross-Cultural Contributions.* New York, N.Y.: Halsted, p. 8; cited in: J. B. Thompson and D. Held (eds.) *Habermas: Critical Debates.* Cambridge, Mass.: The MIT Press, 1982. 70.

Davidson, S. M., and T. R. Marmor. 1980. *The Cost of Living Longer.* Lexington, Mass.: Lexington Books.

Dobrof, R., and E. Litwak. 1977. *Maintenance of Family Ties of Long-Term Care Patients: Theory and Guide to Practice.* Washington, D.C.: National Institute of Mental Health, USGPO, DHEW Publication No. (ADM) 77-400.

Dowd, J. J. 1980. *Stratification Among the Aged.* Monterey, Calif.: Brooks/Cole Publishing Co.

Dowd, J. J., and V. L. Bengtson. 1978. "Aging in Minority Populations: An Examination of the the Double Jeopardy Hypothesis." *Journal of Gerontology* 33: 427–436.

Estes, C. L. 1979. *The Aging Enterprise.* San Francisco, Calif.: Jossey-Bass.

Federal Council on the Aging. 1981. *The Need for Long Term Care: Information and Issues.* Washington, D.C.: United States Government Printing Office.

Feller, B. A. 1983. *Americans Needing Help to Function at Home.* National Center for Health Statistics. *Advance Data from Vital and Health Statistics.* No. 92. DHHS Pub. No. (PHS) 83-1250. Public Health Service, Hyattsville, Md.

Ferlanger, B. 1977. *Natural Helping Networks for the Elderly.* New York, N.Y.: Community Council of Greater New York. Research Utilization Briefs.

Ferraro, K. F. 1980. "Self-Ratings of Health Among the Old and the Old-Old." *Journal of Health and Social Behavior* 21:377–83.

FitzGerald, F. 1983. "Interlude." *The New Yorker,* April 25:54–05.

Folger, J. K., and C. B. Nam. 1967. *Education of the American Population.* Washington, D.C.: U.S. Government Printing Office.

Fontana, A. 1977. *The Last Frontier: The Social Meaning of Growing Old.* Beverly Hills, Calif.: Sage Publications.

Fries, B. E., and L. M. Cooney, Jr. 1985. "Resource Utilization Groups, A Patient Classification System for Long-term Care." *Medical Care* 23 (2).

Fuchs, V. R. 1986. "Sex Differences in Economic Well-being." *Science* 232 (4749): 459–464.

Gelfand, D. E., and A. J. Kutzik (eds.) 1979. *Ethnicity and Aging.* New York, N.Y.: Springer Publishing Co.

George, L. K. 1980. *Role Transitions in Later Life.* Monterey, Calif.: Brooks/Cole Publishing Co.

Gibson, R. C. 1986. "Older Black Americans." *Generations* X (4):35–39.

Gibson, R. M., D. R. Waldo, and K. R. Levit. 1983. "National Health Expenditures, 1982" *Health Care Financing Review* 1 No. 1:1–31.

Glick, P. C. 1977. "Updating the Life Cycle of the Family." *Journal of Marriage and the Family* 39:5–13.

Gouldner, A. W. 1970. *The Coming Crisis of Western Sociology.* New York, N.Y.: Basic Books.

Government Accounting Office. 1977. *The Well-being of Older People in Cleveland Ohio.* Washington, D.C.: Comptroller General of the United States, HRD-77-70.

Grad, S. 1984. "Income of the Population 55 and Over." Social Security Administration, Washington, D.C.: U.S. Government Printing Office.

Grundmann, H. F. 1985. "Adult Programs under the Social Security Act." *Social Security Bulletin* 10:10–21.

Harrington, M. 1962. *The Other America: Poverty in the United States.* New York, N.Y.: Macmillan.

———. 1984. *The New American Poverty.* New York, N.Y.: Penguin Books.

Harvard Medicare Project. 1986. "Medicare: Coming of Age, A Proposal for Reform." Center for Health Policy and Management, John F. Kennedy School of Government, Harvard University, Cambridge, Mass. mimeo.

Havighurst, R. J., and R. Albrecht, 1953. *Older People.* New York, N.Y.: Longmans, Green.

Hochschild, A. 1975. "Disengagement Theory: A Critique and Proposal." *American Sociological Review* 40:553–569.

Holden, K. C., R. V. Burkhauser, and D. A. Myers. 1986. "Income Transitions at Older Stages of Life: The Dynamics of Poverty." *The Gerontologist* 3:292–297.

House, J. S. 1974. "Occupational Stress and Coronary Heart Disease: A Review and Theoretical Integration." *Journal of Health and Social Behavior* 15:12–27.

Jackson, J. J. 1982. "Death Rates of Aged Blacks and Whites, United States, 1964–1978." *The Black Scholar,* 13:36–48.

———. 1985. "Race, National Origin, Ethnicity, and Aging." *In* E. Shanas and R. H. Binstock (eds.), *Handbook of Aging and the Social Sciences (2nd ed.),* New York, N.Y.: Van Nostrand.

Johnson, C. L., and L. A. Grant. 1985. *The Nursing Home in American Society.* Baltimore, Md.: The John Hopkins University Press.

Kahn, A. L. 1987. "Characteristics of Supplementary Security Income Recipients, December 1985." *Social Security Bulletin,* 5:23–57.

Kane, R. A., and R. L. Kane. 1981. *Assessing the Elderly, A Practical Guide to Measurement.* Lexington, Mass: Lexington Books.

Kane, R. L., and R. A. Kane. 1980. "Alternatives to Institutional Care of the Elderly: Beyond the Dichotomy." *The Gerontologist* 20 (3):249–260.

Kastenbaum, R., and S. E. Candy. 1973. "The four percent fallacy: A methodological and empirical critique of extended care facility population statistics." *International Journal of Aging and Human Development* 4:15–21.

Katz, S., T. D. Downs, H. R. Cash, and R. C. Grotz. 1970. "Progress in the Development of the Index of ADL." *Gerontologist* 10(1):20–30.

Katz, S., A. B. Ford, R. W. Moskowitz, B. Jackson, and M. W. Jaffe. 1963. "Studies of Illness in the Aged." *Journal of American Medical Association* 185:914–919.

Keller, T. W. 1985. *Marx's Truth and Its Consequences.* Daly City, Calif.: Prismatique Publications.

Kovar, M. G. 1983. "Expenditures for the medical care of elderly people living in the community throughout 1980." National Medical Care Utilization and Expenditure Survey, Data Report No. 4 DHHS Pub. No. (PHS) 84-20000. National Center for Health Statistics, Public Health Service, Washington D.C. Government Printing Office.

Kuhn, T. S. 1970. *The Structure of Scientific Revolutions, Second Edition, Enlarged.* Chicago. Ill.: The University of Chicago Press.

Kuypers, J. A., and V. L. Bengtson. 1973. "Social Breakdown and Competence." *Human Development* 16:181–201.

Lawton, M. P. 1972. "Assessing the Competence of Older People." *In,* D. P. Kent, R. Kastenbaum, and F. S. Sherwood (eds.) *Research, Planning, and Action for the Elderly.* New York, N.Y.: Behavioral Publications. 122–43.

Lawton, M. P., and E. M. Brody. 1969. "Assessment of Older People: Self-Maintaining and Instrumental Activities of Daily Living."

Lewis, O. 1961. *The Children of Sanchez,* New York, N.Y.: Random House.

Lt. Governor Leo McCarthy's Task Force on the Feminization of Poverty. 1985. *The Feminization of Poverty: Issues and Answers.* Sacramento, Calif.

Lloyd, S., and N. T. Greenspan. 1985. "Nursing Homes, Home Health Services, and Adult Day Care." *In* R. J. Vogel and H. C. Palmer (eds.) *Long-term Care.* Rockville, Md.: Aspen System Corporation.

Lopata, H. Z. 1973. *Widowhood in an American City.* Cambridge, Mass.: Sheckman Publishing Co.

———. 1979. *Women as Widows.* New York, N.Y.: Elsevier Publishing Co.

Louis Harris and Associates. 1986. "Problems Facing Elderly Americans Living Alone." Conducted for the Commonwealth Fund Commission on Elderly People Living Alone. New York, N.Y., mimeo.

Lowenthal, M. F., M. Thurnher, and D. Chiriboga. 1975. *Four Stages of Life.* San Francisco, Calif.: Jossey-Bass.

Lubben, J. E. 1984. "Health and Psychosocial Assessments of Community Based Long Term Care: The California Multipurpose Senior Services Project Experiences, Parts I and II." Berkeley: MSSP Evaluation, University Extension, University of California, Berkeley, mimeo.

———. 1985. "The Relationship of Widowhood, Social Networks and Health to Life Satisfaction Among Poor Elderly Men and Women." School of Social Work, University of California, Los Angeles, mimeo.

Maddox, G. L., and D. C. Dellinger. 1978. "Assessment of Functional Status in a Program Evaluation and Resource Allocation Model." *Annals of the American Academy of Political and Social Science* 438:59–70.

McMillan, A., P. L. Pine, M. Gornick, and R. Prihoda. 1983. "A Study of the 'Crossover Population': Aged Persons Entitled to Both Medicare and Medicaid." *Health Care Financing Review* 4:19–45.

Mechanic, D. 1979. "Correlates of Physician Utilization: Why Do Major Multivariate Studies of Physician Utilization Find Trivial Psychosocial and Organizational Effects?" *Journal of Health and Social Behavior* 20 (December): 387–96.

Menefee, J. A., B. Edwards, and S. J. Schieber. 1981. "Analysis of Nonparticipation in the SSI Program." *Social Security Bulletin* 6:3–21.

Miller, L. S., M. L. Clark, and W. F. Clark. 1985. "The Comparative Evaluation of California's Multipurpose Senior Services Project." *Home Health Care Services Quarterly* VI (3):49–79.

Miller, L. S., *et al.* 1984. "The Comparative Evaluation of California's Multipurpose Senior Services Project: Final Report, 1981–1982." Berkeley: MSSP Evaluation, University Extension, University of California, Berkeley, mimeo.

Miller, R. H. 1982. "Preliminary Report on the Prices of Referred Services." Berkeley: MSSP Evaluation, University Extention, University of California, Berkeley, mimeo.

Minkler, M., and S. R. Blum. 1982. "Community-Based Home Health and Social Services for California's Elderly: Present Constraints and Future Alternatives." Berkeley, California: Institute for Governmental Studies, University of California, Berkeley.

Minkler, M., and C. L. Estes. 1984. *Readings in the Political Economy of Aging.* Farmingdale, N.Y.: Baywood Publishing Company, Inc.

Morgan, L. A. 1986. "The Financial Experience of Widowed Women: Evidence from the LRHA." *The Gerontologist* 6:663–668.

Morris, M. B. 1977. *An Excursion into Creative Sociology.* New York, N.Y.: Columbia University Press.

Moynihan, D. P. 1965. *The Negro Family, The Case for National Action.* Washington, D.C.: U.S. Department of Labor.

Muse, D. N. and D. Sawyer. 1982. *The Medicare and Medicaid Data Book, 1981.* Washington, D.C.: Health Care Financing Administration, Department of Health and Human Services.

Myers, G. C. 1985. "Aging and Worldwide Population Change." *In* E. Shanas and R. H. Binstock (eds.), *Handbook of Aging and the Social Sciences* (2nd ed.), New York: Van Nostrand.

National Center for Health Statistics. 1973. *Net Differences in Interview Data on Chronic Conditions and Information Derived from Medical Records.* HSMHA Publication No. 73-1331, Rockville, Md.

———. 1979. *The National Nursing Home Survey: 1977 Summary for the United States. Vital and Health Statistics,* Series 13, No. 43. Washington, D.C.: United States Government Printing Office.

——. 1984. *Health, United States. 1984.* DHHS Pub. No. (PHS) 85-1232. Public Health Service. Washington, D.C.: United States Government Printing Office.

Nagi, S. 1969. *Disability and Rehabilitation.* Cleveland, Ohio: Ohio State University Press.

National Council on the Aging, Inc. 1981. *Aging in the Eighties: America in Transition* (Louis Harris and Associates, Inc.) Washington, D.C.: National Council on the Aging, Inc.

Neugarten, B. L. 1968. *Middle Age and Aging.* Chicago, Ill.: University of Chicago Press.

Palmore, E. 1976. "Total Chance of Institutionalization among the Aged." *Gerontologist* 16:504–507.

Paterson, J. T. 1981. *America's Struggle Against Poverty, 1900–1980.* Cambridge, Mass.: Harvard University Press.

Pearce, D. 1978. "The Feminization of Poverty: Women, Work and Welfare." *Urban & Social Change* 11:28–36.

Pearce, D., and H. McAdoo. 1981. *Women and Children: Alone and in Poverty.* Center for National Policy Review, Catholic University Law School, Washington, D.C.

Pelham, A. O. 1980. Plainsclothes Investigator in Cockroach Castles. Ph.D. Dissertation, Department of Sociology, University of California, San Francisco.

Pelham, A. O., and W. F. Clark. 1982. "When Do You Go Home? Hospital Discharge and Placement Decisions for the Elderly and Implications for Community-based Long-term Care Agencies." Paper presented at the 110th Annual meeting of the American Public Health Association, November 14–18, Montreal, Quebec, Canada.

——. 1983. Widowhood Among Low Income Ethnic Minorities in California. Paper presented at the 29th Annual Meeting of the Western Gerontological Society, Albuquerque, New Mexico, April 16.

——. 1986a. "Interviewing Challenges of the California Senior Survey." *In,* A. O. Pelham and W. F. Clark (eds.), *Managing Home Care for the Elderly.* New York, N.Y.: Springer Publishing Co.

——. 1986b. "Introduction." *In,* A. O. Pelham, and W. F. Clark (eds.), *Managing Home Care for the Elderly.* New York, N.Y.: Springer Publishing Co.

——. 1986c. 'Social Policy Implications of the Community-Based Long-Term Care Experiences." In, A. O. Pelham and W. F. Clark (eds.), *Managing Home Care for the Elderly.* New York, N.Y.: Springer Publishing Company.

Pfeiffer, E. 1975. "A Short Portable Mental Status Questionnaire for the Assessment of Organic Brain Deficit in Elderly Patients." *Journal of the American Geriatrics Society* XXIII: 433–441.

Phillips, B. S. 1957. "A Role Theory Approach to Adjustment in Old Age." *American Sociological Review* 22:212–217.

President's National Advisory Council on Economic Opportunity. 1981. *Final Report—The American Promise: Equal Justice and Economic Opportunity.* Washington, D.C.: National Advisory Council, 13th Annual Report: 46.

Preston, S. H. 1984. "Children and the Elderly in the U.S." *Scientific American* 251 (6):44–49.

Rich, B. M., and M. Baum. 1984. *The Aging: A Guide to Public Policy*. Pittsburgh, Pa.: University of Pittsburgh Press.

Riley, M. W. 1971. "Social Gerontology and Age Stratification of Society." *Gerontologist* 11:79–87.

Rose, A. M. 1965. "The Subculture of the Aging: A Framework for Research in Social Gerontology." *In*, A. M. Rose and W. Peterson (eds.), *Older People and Their Social Worlds*. Philadelphia, Pa.: F. A. Davis Co.

Rosenmayr, L., and E. Köckeis. 1963. "Propositions for a Sociological Theory of Aging and the Family." *International Social Science Journal* XV: 410–426.

Rosenwaike, I. 1985. "A Demographic Portrait of the Oldest Old." *Milbank Memorial Fund Quarterly/Health and Society* 2:187–205.

Rosow, I. 1974. *Socialization to Old Age*. Berkeley, Calif.: University of California Press.

Rubin, M. 1981. "Women and Poverty." Washington, D.C.: Business and Professional Women's Foundation.

Sangl, J. A. 1985. "The Family Support System of the Elderly," In R. J. Vogel and H. C. Palmer (eds.) *Long-term Care*. Rockville, Md.: Aspen System Corp.

Schatzman, L. 1982. Professor of Sociology, University of California, San Francisco. Personal Communication.

Scherf, B. A. 1982. "Interrater Reliability: Initial Assessment Instruments." Sacramento: California Health and Welfare Agency, MSSP Working Paper, No. 4A, mimeo.

———. 1983. "Interrater Reliability: Revised Instruments." Sacramento: California Health and Welfare Agency, MSSP Working Paper, No. 4B, mimeo.

Schulz, J. H. 1985. *The Economics of Aging, Third Edition,* New York, N.Y.: Van Nostrand Reinhold Co.

Shanas, E. 1977. *National Survey of the Aged*. Final Report to the Administration on Aging. Grant No. 90-A-369.

———. 1979a "Social Myth as Hypothesis: The Case of Family Relations of Old People." *Gerontologist* 19 (Issue 1, February): 3–9.

———. 1979b "The Family as a Social Support System in Old Age." *Gerontologist* 19 (Issue 2, April): 169–174.

Shanas, E., and G. L. Maddox. 1985. "Health, Health Resources, and the Utilization of Care." *In*, E. Shanas and R. H. Binstock (eds.), *Handbook of Aging and the Social Sciences* (2nd ed.), New York, N.Y.: Van Nostrand.

Sheldon, J. H. 1948. *The Social Medicine of Old Age: Report of an Inquiry in Wolverhampton*. London: Oxford University Press. Reprinted by Arno Press, New York, N.Y., 1980.

Silverstone, B. 1985. "Informal Social Support Systems for the Frail Elderly." *In*, Committee on an Aging Society, Institute of Medicine and National Research Council, *America's Aging: Health in an Older Society*. Washington, D.C.: National Academy Press.

Smeeding, T. M. 1982. "Alternative Methods for Valuing Selected In-kind Transfer Benefits and Measuring Their Effect on Poverty." Technical Paper 50. Washington, D.C.: U.S. Bureau of the Census.

Social Security Bulletin. 1986. Vol. 49, no. 3:3.

Steinem, G. 1983. *Outrageous Acts and Everyday Rebellions*. New York: Holt Rinehart and Winston.

Stone, R., G. L. Cafferata, and J. Sangl. 1986. *Caregivers of the Frail Elderly: A National Profile.* Rockville, Md.: National Center for Health Services Research.

Sussman, M. B. 1985. "The Family Life of Old People." *In,* E. Shanas and R. H. Binstock (eds.), *Handbook of Aging and the Social Sciences (2nd ed.),* New York, N.Y.: Van Nostrand.

Suzman, R., and M. W. Riley. 1985. "Introducing the 'Oldest Old.'" *Milbank Memorial Fund Quarterly/Health and Society* 2:177–186.

Tissue, T. 1978. *A Last Look at Adult Welfare Recipients Prior to SSI.* Washington, D.C.: Office of Research and Statistics, Social Security Administration. HEW Publication No. (SSA) 78–11723.

Tobin, S. S., and M. A. Lieberman. 1976. *Last Home for the Aged.* San Francisco, Calif.: Jossey-Bass.

Torres-Gil, F. (1986) "An Examination of Factors Affecting Future Cohorts of Elderly Hispanics." *Gerontologist* 26: 140–146.

Tuma, N. B., and L. D. Groeneveld. 1979. "Dynamic analysis of event histories," *American Journal of Sociology* 84:820–54.

Uehara, E. S., S. Geron, and S. K. Beeman. 1986. "The Elderly Poor in the Reagan era." *Gerontologist* 1:48–55.

United States Bureau of the Census. 1978–79. Current Population Reports, Special Studies, Series P-23, No. 85. *Social and Economic Characteristics of the Older Population: 1978.* Washington, D.C.: U.S. Government Printing Office.

———. 1981. Current Population Reports, Series P-20, no. 365. *Marital Status and Living Arrangements: March 1980.* Washington, D.C.: U.S. Government Printing Office.

———. 1981. Supplementary Reports, PC 80-S1-1. *Age, Sex, Race, and Spanish Origin of the Population by Regions, Divisions, and States: 1980.* Washington, D.C.: U.S. Government Printing Office.

———. 1983a. Current Population Reports, Series P-23, no. 124. *Child Support and Alimony: 1981 (Advance Report).* Washington, D.C.: U.S. Government Printing Office.

———. 1983b. Current Population Reports, Series P-23, no. 128. *America in Transition: An Aging Society.* Washington, D.C.: U.S. Government Printing Office.

———. 1983c. Current Population Reports, P-60, no. 143. *Characteristics of Households and Persons Receiving Selected Noncash Benefits: 1982.* Washington, D.C.: U.S. Government Printing Office.

———. 1983d. *General Population Characteristics, United States Summary, 1980 Census of Population.* Volume 1, chapter B, Part 1, PC80-1-B1, Table 41.

———. 1984a. Current Population Reports, P-60, no. 144. *Characteristics of the Population below the Poverty Level: 1982.* Washington, D.C.: U.S. Government Printing Office.

———. 1984b. Current Population Reports, Series P-60, no. 145. *Money Income and Poverty Status of Families and Persons in the United States: 1983 (Advance Data from the March 1984 Current Population Survey),* Washington, D.C.: U.S. Government Printing Office.

———. 1985a. Current Population Reports, March 1985, P-60, no. 152. *Money Income and Poverty Status of Families and Persons in the United States: 1984.* Washington, D.C.: U.S. Government Printing Office.

———. 1985b. Current Population Reports, P-60, no. 147. *Characteristics of the Population below the Poverty Level: 1983.* Washington, D.C.: U.S. Government Printing Office.

———. 1985c. Current Population Reports, March 1985, P-60, no. 149. *Money Income and Poverty Status of Families and Persons in the United States: 1984.* Washington, D.C.: U.S. Government Printing Office.

———. 1987a. Current Population Reports. P-60, no. 155. *Receipt of Selected Noncash Benefits: 1985.* Washington, D.C.: U.S. Government Printing Office.

———. 1987b. Current Population Reports. P-60, no. 157. *Money Income and Poverty Status of Families and Persons in the United States: 1986.* Washington, D.C.: U.S. Government Printing Office.

U.S. Congress. 1980. *Report of the 1979 Advisory Council on Social Security.* U.S. House of Representatives, Committee on Ways and Means, Washington, D.C.: U.S. Government Printing Office.

———. 1982. *Developments in Aging: 1981.* Washington, D.C.: Special Committee on Aging, United States Senate, Report 97–314, Vol. 1.

———. 1984. *Developments in Aging: 1983.* Washington, D.C.: Special Committee on Aging, United States Senate, Report 98–360, Vol. 2.

———. 1985. *America in Transition: An Aging Society, 1984–85 Edition.* Washington, D.C.: Special Committee on Aging, United States Senate. Washington, D.C.: U.S. Government Printing Office.

———. 1986a. *Background Material and Data on Programs within the Jurisdiction of the Committee on Ways and Means.* Committee on Ways and Means, United States House of Representatives, 99th Congress, 2nd Session. Washington, D.C.: U.S. Government Printing Office.

———. 1986b. *Nursing Home Care: The Unfinished Agenda.* Special Committee on Aging, United States Senate, Serial No. 99-J. Washington, D.C.: U.S. Government Printing Office.

———. 1986c. *The Impact of Gramm-Rudman-Hollings on Programs Serving Older Americans.* Washington, D.C.: Special Committee on Aging, United States Senate. Washington, D.C.: U.S. Government Printing Office.

United States Department of Health and Human Services. (1984). *Program and Demographic Characteristics of Supplemental Security Income Beneficiaries, December 1983.* Social Security Administration (SSA Publication No. 13-11977), Washington, D.C.: U.S. Government Printing Office.

United States Department of Health, Education, and Welfare. 1977. *Characteristics, Social Contacts, and Activities of Nursing Home Residents.* Washington, D.C.: U.S. Government Printing Office. National Center for Health Statistics, Vital and Health Statistics, Series 13, No. 27.

———. 1981. *Characteristics of Nursing Home Residents, Health Status, and Care Received: National Nursing Home Survey, United States, May-December 1977.* National Center for Health Statistics, Vital and Health Statistics, Series 13, No. 51. Washington, D.C.: U.S. Government Printing Office.

United States Department of Labor, Bureau of Labor Statistics. 1966. *Retired Couple's Budget for a Moderate Living Standard.* Bulletin No. 1570-4. Washington, D.C.: U.S. Government Printing Office.

————. 1982a. *The Female-Male Earnings Gap: A Review of Employment and Earnings Issues.* Washington, D.C.: U.S. Government Printing Office.

————. 1982b. "Retired Couple's Budgets, Final Report, Autumn 1981." *Monthly Labor Review,* 105 (November): 37–38.

Villers Foundation. 1987. *On the Other Side of Easy Street.* Washington, D.C.: The Villers Foundation.

Vladeck, B. C. 1980. *Unloving Care.* New York, N.Y.: Basic Books, Inc.

Vogel, R. J., and H. C. Palmer, (eds.). 1985. *Long-term Care.* Rockville, Md.: Aspen System Corp.

Wan, T. T. H., W. G. Weissert, and B. B. Livieratos. 1980. "Geriatric Day Care and Homemaker Services: An Experimental Study." *Journal of Gerontology* 35 (2):256–74.

Warlick, J. L. 1985. "Why is Poverty After 65 a Woman's Problem?" *Journal of Gerontology* 40 (6):751–757.

Warski, W., and D. Green. 1971. "Evaluation in a Home-Care Program." *Medical Care* 9:352–364.

Wershow, H. J. 1976. "The Four Percent Fallacy." *Gerontologist* 16:52–55.

Wood, V., M. Wylie, and B. Shaefor. 1969. "An Analysis of a Short Self-Report Measure of Life Satisfaction: Correlation with Rater Judgment." *Journal of Gerontology* 24(4):465–469.

Wright, K. 1974. "Alternative Measures of the Output of Social Programmes: The Elderly." *In,* A. Culyer, (ed.) *Economics Policies and Social Goals.* London: Martin Robertson and Co., Ltd.

Wylie, C., and B. White. 1964. "A Measure of Disability." *Archives of Environmental Health* 8:834–39.

Zedlewski, S. R., and J. A. Meyer. 1987. "Toward Ending Poverty among the Elderly and Disabled: Policy and Financing Options." Washington, D.C.: The Urban Institute.

Zick, C. D. and K. R. Smith. 1986. "Immediate and Delayed Effects of Widowhood on Poverty: Patterns from the 1970s." *Gerontologist* 6:669–675.

Index

About the Authors

William F. Clark, M.P.P., served in the Peace Corps in Peru for eight years before entering graduate school. After receiving his degree in public policy from the University of California, Berkeley, in 1976, he continued public service with the State of California. Currently, he is employed by the San Francisco State University Foundation, Inc. Mr. Clark has written on widowhood among low-income elderly and their informal support systems, and is coauthor of *Managing Home Care for the Elderly*. He is also an instructor at San Francisco State University, where he teaches aging policy courses. Mr. Clark's primary research is in the delivery of services to low-income elders. He also retains his interest in pre-Columbian art and cultures.

Anabel O. Pelham, Ph. D., is currently Professor and Director of Gerontology Programs at San Francisco State University. She received her degree from the University of California, San Francisco. Her professional experiences include academic and older adult education program development, teaching in interdisciplinary gerontology, university administration, and research. Dr. Pelham has written on medical sociology, qualitative methods in field research, aging policy, and theory and gerontology, and is coauthor of *Managing Home Care for the Elderly*. She is a member of the Board of Directors and president-elect of the California Council of Gerontology and Geriatrics. She is also a member of the Board of Directors of Northern California Presbyterian Homes. Her current research interests include aging social policy, the social construction of aging, and applied gerontology. Dr. Pelham resides in San Francisco and is a collector of northern California red wines.

Marleen L. Clark, D.S.W., received her graduate education at the University of California, Berkeley, where her primary areas of interest were research, economics, and the administration of social services. Dr. Clark is presently Research Manager of PACE, On Lok Senior Services' national replication project for care of the frail elderly. Her professional activities have included research on the equity of distribution in in-home services and implementation of an information system to increase the fairness of awards. She was Assistant Director for the Evaluation Unit for California's Multipurpose Senior Services Program, where her area of research was medical costs. She helped to establish a software firm, Berkeley System Design, and was instrumental in the development of a software program to facilitate use of personal computers by the visually handicapped.